# asSALTed

### Saving Lives and Money
### by Adopting the Finnish Salt Laws

**Guido Filler, MD, PhD, FRCPC**
**Professor of Paediatrics**

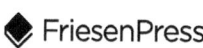 FriesenPress

Suite 300 - 990 Fort St
Victoria, BC, V8V 3K2
Canada

www.friesenpress.com

ISBN
978-1-5255-6996-8 (Hardcover)
978-1-5255-6997-5 (Paperback)
978-1-5255-6998-2 (eBook)

*1. HEALTH & FITNESS, NUTRITION*

Distributed to the trade by The Ingram Book Company

# Table of Contents

# Preface

Are you aware of this alarming fact? The incidence of kidney stones is increasing, and it's likely because of the salt in our diets. You can even get this painful condition several times over your lifetime. In the past, kidney stones were most common in old men. Now, it's become rampant among teenagers. And that's alarming because kidney stones may also cause kidney failure and a shorter life expectancy! But it is preventable.

How do I know this? Because kidneys are my specialty. I am a kidney doctor for children (what we call a "paediatric nephrologist"). Today we're also finding an increase of kidney stones in children, and especially in adolescent girls. One of the roles of a kidney doctor for children is to prevent new stones. **This book is my call to action!**

So what is the solution? We've seen in Finnish studies that reducing salt intake by 40% can substantially reduce disease and deaths due to high blood pressure. This is profound! Low salt diets are also associated with a lower risk of kidney stones, osteoporosis (bone loss), obesity, chronic kidney disease, cataracts and macular degeneration.

As a kidney doctor, I see children with kidney stones daily. Most often, these children are otherwise completely healthy. Even more disturbing is the fact that every five years the number of children and adolescents with kidney stones doubles. It's heartbreaking to see these young people suffer through the worst pain known to humankind as they pass a stone. It also concerns me that, in most cases, the stones occur because of what these children and adolescents are eating. A diet high in salt and protein, and low in vegetables and water, forms the perfect storm for creating a condition that we used to only see in older people. Let's heal our bodies. Let's protect our children and ourselves!

## How Kidney Stones Form

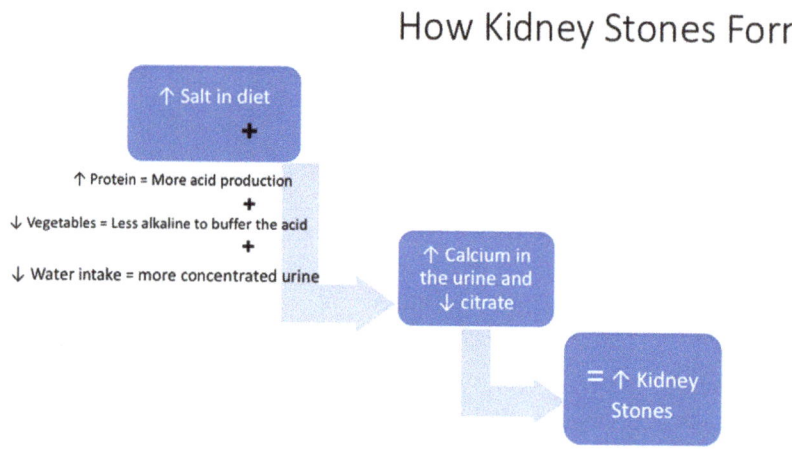

**Figure 1:** *Simple diagram of kidney stone formation*

All of us eat a lot of salty food—on average 3,700 mg of salt per day—but our sodium intake should be less than 2,000 mg per day. We eat almost twice the amount of salt we should be eating! A high-salt diet leads to calcium wasting in the urine. For children's bone health, this is a problem as they may not reach their peak bone mass because of this preventable calcium wasting.

If you add to a salty diet a lot of protein, little or no vegetables, and little water intake, the amount of calcium in your urine increases. The more salt you eat, the more salt your kidneys need to remove. The more salt that gets in the urine, the less calcium can be reabsorbed and gets wasted in the urine. Having a lot of calcium in the urine promotes stones.

It's puzzling that today's youth, especially adolescent girls, are affected. Normally, we see more citrate in the urine of adolescent girls than in the urine of adolescent boys. Citrate envelopes calcium (binding it and reducing the amount of calcium available for stone formation), so girls *should* have a lower chance of getting kidney stones. At all other ages, males form more kidney stones than females.

We don't yet fully understand the reason for this rapid increase of kidney stones in adolescent girls. One of my patients gave me this explanation: "Girls are more petite but are more focused on how they look. They eat less of everything, including water." If adolescent girls eat the same portions as teenage boys in fast food restaurants, girls are actually eating more salt per body weight. Indeed, more than 75% of the salt we eat is in processed food and fast food. Unfortunately, it's often cheaper than healthy food, which means many people with low incomes are inadvertently encouraged to eat an unhealthy diet.

Our youth today are eating about 12 times more salt than those in the 1970s. This is staggering since salt is linked to so many diseases. I mentioned our kidney stone epidemic to my friend Christer Holmberg, a paediatric nephrologist from Helsinki, Finland. He replied, "Kidney stones? We don't see kidney stones in our population."

That made me curious. I then learned about the 1972 anti-salt campaign in Finland's province of North Karelia. This campaign went viral, leading to a 40% reduction of salt intake across the country. The impact of these changes is profound. Strokes were reduced by 82%. Heart attacks were reduced by 75%. Hip fractures caused by osteoporosis dropped by 50%. The most profound result of the campaign was that legislation was passed to control the amount of salt in processed food. The Finnish government can fine businesses if they put too much salt in food. The government also worked with the food industry to look at suitable potassium-based salt alternatives.

We need to stop poisoning ourselves with too much salt and enjoy healthier and longer lives. We need to decrease conditions such as heart disease, high blood pressure, dementia, stroke, heart attacks, cataracts, macular degeneration, chronic kidney disease and obesity. I predict there will be a strong increase of hip and other fractures among our current youth at a much earlier age than what we've seen in past generations.

If I had a magic wand, I would cut everyone's salt intake by half. We can only do that if we crack down on the restaurant and food-processing industries and hold them accountable. Reducing salt intake would also dramatically free up billions of health care dollars. We just need to look at Finland to learn about the incredible health benefits of reducing salt. Without regulation and legislation from government, the downward trend of life expectancy will continue, and health care will become more expensive for all of us. We need to help advocate for much stricter salt laws.

The life expectancy in North America is declining for the third year in a row. As a father of four children and grandfather of two grandchildren, this concerns me. I want my children and grandchildren to live far longer than I ever will.

Guido Filler, MD, PhD, FRCPC
Professor of Paediatrics
London, Ontario, December 2019

# Introduction

In the last 50 years, humankind has reached outer space, developed driverless cars and transformed global communication. We've eradicated smallpox with vaccinations and cut down diseases like tuberculosis and influenza. We've even made progress with the treatment of cancer, heart disease and stroke—the three biggest killers today. Yet despite all our medical and technological advances, life expectancy is steadily declining in North America.[1] And it's declining at a rate unlike anything we've seen since World War I and the Spanish influenza.[2]

The World Health Organization (WHO) lists Italy as the healthiest country in the world, followed by Iceland, Switzerland, Singapore and Australia. Canada ranks 17. The United States is not among the top 25 nations.[3] The healthiest nations by population are Japan, Germany, the United Kingdom, France and Italy. So, why is the United States not among the top 25 nations? What on earth is going on?

This book is an example of what happens when science, research and health professionals decide to cooperate and investigate a mystery. But, rather than the shocking discovery of a single secret killer in our midst, the answer is a little more complicated. It has all the major elements of a good murder mystery novel: political intrigue, opportunistic elements of nature, terrible accidents and cosmically bad decisions.

*AsSALTed* is a warning about the unintended consequences of current North American legislation, or lack thereof, around salt in processed foods. Heart disease may be North America's number one killer by name, but the cause of its declining life-expectancy rates may be salt—a tasty ocean dust.

This book is also a call to action because there is a solution.

*Note: In order for this book to reach the widest audience possible, citations have been moved to the end of the book for flow. There, you'll also find extra information and a wealth of rich resources to satisfy more in-depth investigation. Make sure to check out the Notes section!*

# Chapter 1:
# Current Salt Legislation
# in Developed Countries

Salt—the chemical compound also known as sodium chloride—is usually found in seawater. It's a necessary element in the diet of humans, animals and many plants. It's also necessary for food preservation. Salt has been an important part of the world's history as far back as 6050 BC. The Egyptians used it for religious offerings and as a trade item with the Phoenicians. There are written records of salt use in China that date back as far as 2700 BC. Salt was a major revenue source in trade since it was scarce for a very long time. It has been a major part of economic success in certain civilizations, most notably Venice because of its salt monopoly.[4]

## The World Health Organization declares war on high-salt intake

Sodium is an essential nutrient. Though the main source of sodium is sodium chloride, it can also come from sodium glutamate, which is used as a condiment in many parts of the world. Sodium is needed for normal cell function, transmission of nerve impulses, acid base balance and maintenance of plasma (part of the blood) volume. However, too much sodium is linked to high blood pressure and many other chronic non-communicable diseases.[5] WHO states: "High sodium consumption (more than 2,000 milligrams/day) and insufficient potassium intake (less than 3.5 grams/day) contribute to high blood pressure and increase the risk of heart disease and stroke."[6] However, even less than 2,300 mg would be a major achievement.

WHO also states that an estimated 2.5 million deaths could be prevented each year if salt consumption around the world was reduced to the recommended level (less than 2,300 mg per day).[7] Meanwhile, there's no legislation around salt in food in Canada or in most countries.

It's been found that legal requirements are more effective in reducing salt in processed food than voluntary targets or agreements because violations can be penalized. While all WHO member states agreed in 2013 to reduce the global population's salt consumption by 30% by 2025,[8] very few countries have laws that regulate the salt content in food. Only 38 countries have voluntary or legally binding salt content targets. South Africa and Argentina are among the few countries with legally binding standards across a broad range of processed food. These include bread, cured meats, soups, stock and snack foods. In Argentina, apart from cured meats and sausages, 15 out of 18 food groups showed median values below the targets that were established.[9] There are only seven more countries with legally binding maximum salt levels for at least one product, usually bread,[10] even though salt reduction has been shown to be one of the most cost-effective and, in some cases, cost-saving way of reducing the growing burden of cardiovascular disease and stroke.[11]

The WHO website gives very detailed advice on how to reduce salt in your diet.[12]

## How to reduce salt in diets

Government policies and strategies should create environments that enable populations to consume adequate quantities of safe and nutritious foods that make up a healthy diet including low salt. Improving dietary habits is a societal as well as an individual responsibility. It demands a population-based, multisectoral, and culturally relevant approach.

Key broad strategies for salt reduction include:

- government policies - including appropriate fiscal policies and regulation to ensure food manufacturers and retailers produce healthier foods or make healthy products available and affordable;
- working with the private sector to improve the availability and accessibility of low-salt products;
- consumer awareness and empowerment of populations through social marketing and mobilization to raise awareness of the need to reduce salt intake consumption;
- creating an enabling environment for salt reduction through local policy inter-ventions and the promotion of "healthy food" settings such as schools, workplaces, communities, and cities;
- monitoring of population salt intake, sources of salt in the diet and consumer knowledge, attitudes and behaviours relating to salt to inform policy decisions.

Salt reduction programmes and programmes that promote fortification with micronutrients of salt, condiments or seasonings high in salt (bouillon cubes, soy and fish sauce) can complement each other.

Salt consumption at home can be reduced by:

- not adding salt during the preparation of food;
- not having a salt shaker on the table;
- limiting the consumption of salty snacks;
- choosing products with lower sodium content.

Other local practical actions to reduce salt intake include:

- integrating salt reduction into the training curriculum of food handlers;
- removing salt shakers and soy sauce from tables in restaurants; Introducing product or shelf labels making it clear that certain products are high in sodium;
- providing targeted dietary advice to people visiting health facilities;
- advocating for people to limit their intake of products high in salt and advocating that they reduce the amount of salt used for cooking; and
- educating children and providing a supportive environment for children so that they start early with adopting low salt diets.

Actions by the food industry should include:

- incrementally reducing salt in products over time so that consumers adapt to the taste and don't switch to alternative products;
- promoting the benefits of eating reduced salt foods through consumer awareness activities in food outlets;
- reducing salt in foods and meals served at restaurants and catering outlets and labelling sodium content of foods and meals.

**Figure 2:** *World Health Organization suggestions for reducing salt in your diet.*

## Canada and WHO's call to action

What did Canada do in response to WHO's call to action? It appealed to the food industry to voluntarily reduce salt additives in processed food. It introduced mandatory labelling and definitions for "reduced sodium". Health Canada states that heart disease and stroke are among the leading causes of death at a rate of 55%.[13] On December 14, 2016, new food and drug regulations came into force for nutrition labelling, lists of ingredients, and food colour requirements. There was a five-year transition period to meet the new requirement.[14] In 2017, the Canadian health department analyzed if the food industry was following the lower sodium guideline. Only 14% of the food products met the phase III target and 48% of the food categories didn't take any steps to meet the sodium-reduction target.[15] The result: Reduction of sodium in processed food was very low and did not meet expectations.

| **Nutrition Facts**<br>**Valeur nutritive**<br>Per 1 cup (250 mL)<br>pour 1 tasse (250 mL) | |
|---|---|
| **Calories 110** | **% Daily Value***<br>**% valeur quotidienne*** |
| **Fat / Lipides** 0 g | 0 % |
| Saturated / saturés 0 g<br>+ Trans / trans 0 g | 0 % |
| **Carbohydrate / Glucides** 26 g | |
| Fibre / Fibres 0 g | 0 % |
| Sugars / Sucres 22 g | 22 % |
| **Protein / Protéines** 2 g | |
| **Cholesterol / Cholestérol** 0 mg | |
| **Sodium** 0 mg | 0 % |
| Potassium 450 mg | 10 % |
| Calcium 30 mg | 2 % |
| Iron / Fer 0 mg | 0 % |

*5% or less is **a little**, 15% or more is **a lot**
*5% ou moins c'est **peu**, 15% ou plus c'est **beaucoup**

**Figure 3:** *A typical Canadian nutrition fact label as now required by law. Source: "Information within the nutrition facts table: mandatory information," Canadian Food Inspection Agency, Government of Canada, http://www.inspection.gc.ca/food/requirements-and-guidance/labelling/industry/nutrition-labelling/nutrition-facts-table/eng/1389198568400/1389198597278?chap=1.*

## The US and WHO's call to action

What happened in the United States? In 2006, the American Medical Association brought its salt policy into the headlines. These were its demands: [16]

Urge the Food and Drug Administration (FDA) to revoke the "generally recognized as safe" status of salt and develop regulatory measures limiting the amount of salt in processed and restaurant foods.

Establish quantifiable milestones, specifically a 50% reduction over the next decade, in the salt content of processed foods, fast-food products and restaurant meals.

Join in partnership with organizations to educate consumers about the benefits of long-term salt reduction.

Work with the FDA to improve food labelling and develop warning labels for foods high in salt.

The salt industry's response was swift and predictable and tried to confuse the issue. The government uptake was nil. As late as July 24, 2019, Congress had temporarily blocked the FDA from implementing voluntary industry targets for sodium reduction in processed food. Congress claimed this was for financial reasons.[17]

By contrast, the salt campaign in Finland was highly successful. One of the key differences was legislation.

## Is sea salt better than table salt?

The short answer is "No." While table salt is more heavily processed to eliminate minerals and usually contains an additive to prevent clumping, there is no difference in sodium levels between sea salt and table salt. They have comparable amounts of sodium by weight. Sea salt and table salt have the same basic nutritional value, despite the fact that sea salt is often promoted as a healthier alternative.

Sea salt is produced by evaporating water from the oceans or saltwater lakes, usually with little processing. Depending on the water source, this leaves behind certain trace minerals and elements. The minerals add flavour and colour to sea salt, which also comes in a variety of coarseness levels. There is also iodine in sea salt, which our bodies need. However, the amount of sodium is the same.

## Summary

Most governments have growing awareness about the need to reduce salt in processed food—although they're coming to that awareness three decades later than Finland. All WHO member states joined the 2013 World Health Assembly and signed on to reduce salt intake by 30% in 2025. However, the voluntary measures have not, by and large, been implemented, and there has been no significant progress in the reduction of cardiovascular disease and stroke-related deaths. It may not be possible to achieve the 2025 goals without stricter legislation similar to that of Finland and the other eight nations that regulate salt content in processed food.

# Chapter 2:
# Kidney Stones and Salt

## In agonizing pain

Fifteen-year-old Claudia was in agonizing pain. It felt like someone was stabbing her left side with a knife. She couldn't keep her food down. Her urine looked like blood. The pain moved into her left groin before she suddenly lost consciousness and was rushed to the nearest hospital.

Claudia was dosed with morphine and given an ultrasound. It showed a seven-millimetre stone in her ureter, a tube that connects the left kidney to the bladder. She was given medication intravenously that had a strange metallic taste. The stone was too big to pass so Claudia needed surgery to unblock her kidney. After surgery, Claudia spent several days in the hospital to recover.

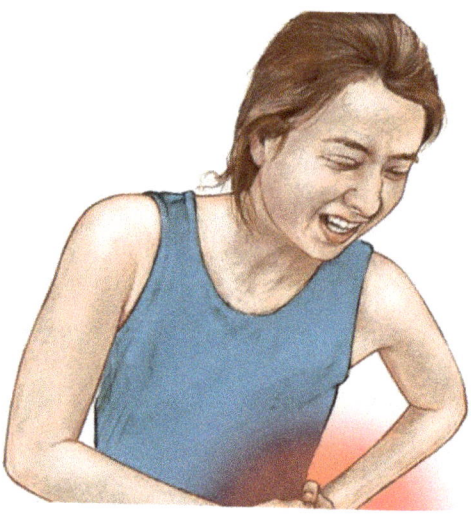

**Figure 4:** *Women report that the pain from kidney stones is similar to the pain of giving birth.*

Claudia was your typical teenager. She was thin, and her nutrition was mostly sugary snacks and fast food. Claudia maintained this diet for some time. She couldn't stand her mom's home-cooked meals. Her favourite snack was potato chips. At home, she also snacked on cheese. Vegetables? No thank you! While her mom was going on about her poor eating habits, Claudia recognized she was underweight and received no nutritional value from meals. These sugary snacks with high-fructose corn starch were irresistible. When she did eat at home, it was mostly meat and cold cuts; she rarely ate fruit, and lemons held no appeal. For fluids, she drank sugary drinks and beverages with a ton of caffeine.

This is the typical diet of the modern teenager. According to American studies, the typical teenager consumes about 3,310 mg of sodium per day.[18] Canadians eat about 3,400 mg of sodium every single day.[19] This is more than double what we need. No one should eat more than 2,000 mg of sodium (one teaspoon of salt) per day.[20]

## Why did Claudia get a kidney stone?

A few weeks later, Claudia saw a kidney specialist for a workup of her kidney stones. The goal was to prevent new stones from forming.[21] The ultrasound showed another stone in the left kidney; her urologist had told her she had a 50% chance of getting another one. The kidney doctor asked what her diet was like and did a test that required plenty of urine. She went back a few weeks later for her results.

At the follow-up visit, the kidney doctor told her that her urine composition promotes stone formation, and she would be at risk for more stones if she didn't make changes to her diet. The good news was that lifestyle changes were enough to keep her from getting more stones. She would have to eat less salt and more vegetables and drink two litres (or two quarts) of water each day.

If you are a kidney stone patient, you should have a low salt intake, but it's not easy. Eighty percent of the salt we consume is in processed food—only 10% is added during cooking and 10% is table salt. For Canadians, the foods that contribute most to our sodium intake are breads (14%), processed meats (9%) and pasta dishes (6%). The rate for breads is higher mainly because we eat more of it, rather than it having more sodium.[22] It's actually impossible to have a low-salt diet if you don't give up processed food.

Claudia hated the taste of water and decided to ignore the doctor's advice. She was back in the emergency room three months later and ended up being put on chronic medication with potassium citrate. Eventually, she changed her diet, and she was able to stop taking medication a few years later.

Claudia's story is typical. It is heard repeatedly, three to five times per week every single week of the year, by every single paediatric kidney specialist in the country. The rate of kidney stones in adolescent children is literally doubling every five years.[23] Kidney stones are a chronic disease.[24] Almost half of these children suffer more stones over several months or years. But we rarely find it's genetic (inherited from family).[25] Most of these children have never had kidney infections before, and we don't find structural anomalies in their kidneys. That's good news because it means kidney stones *are* lifestyle related and can be prevented.

## Kidney stones are a public health issue

Kidney stones have traditionally been the disease of older men.[26] By the age of 70, we see kidney stones in 11% of adult men and 6% of adult women.[27] However, patients are getting younger and younger. Even among children and adolescents, we're seeing significantly more kidney stones, especially in teenage girls.[28]

Often, kidney stones are small enough to pass without major treatment. However, passing kidney stones ranks as the most excruciating pain known to human beings. Some women have said the pain is worse than giving birth. Over the last several decades, we've seen more existing cases and new cases, and after you've had an initial stone, you're more likely to form another one. The influence of diet on the risk for kidney stones cannot be overstated. Kidney stones place a significant burden on the health care system, and this is likely to increase with time.[29]

Let's look at some data in the United States for the years 1992, 1998 and 2000.[30]

**Table 2-1:** Comparisons of US data

|  | 1992 | 2000 |
| --- | --- | --- |
| Kidney stone rate | 71 per 100,000 people | 184 per 100,000 people |
| Outpatient visits | 950,000 | 1,825,000 |
|  | **1998** | **2000** |
| Male-to-female ratio | 1.86 | 1.45 |
| Average length of hospital stay | 2 days | 3 days |
|  | **1992** | **1998** |
| Visit rates for kidney stones | 123 per 100,000 visits | 199 per 100,000 visits |

- In 1992, the overall kidney stone rate was 71 per 100,000 people; it rose to 184 per 100,000 people in 2000.[31] Outpatient visits nearly doubled during this time, from 950,000 in 1992 to 1.8 million in 2000.
- In 1998, more males were hospitalized, but the male-to-female ratio decreased from 1.86 in 1998 to 1.45 in 2000. This likely reflects an increase in females being hospitalized. The average length of stay was two days in 1998 and three days in 2000.
- In 1998, there were 66,580 surgeries in an ambulatory surgery centre. That year, the visit rate for kidney stones rose from 123 per 100,000 visits in 1992 to 199 per 100,000 visits. In 1998, treatments included shock-wave lithotripsy (54%), ureteroscopy (41%) and removal with surgery (4%). Patients also often required medications.
- In 2000, visits to the emergency room totalled 617,647 with an overall rate of 226 visits for kidney stones per 100,000. Males visited the emergency room twice as much as females. For outpatient hospital and clinic visits, the rate of kidney stones was 731 per 100,000.
- In all years, Caucasians had the highest rate of hospitalization.[32]

## We are getting kidney stones earlier in life

People are getting their first kidney stones at younger ages. In children, there has been a substantial increase in kidney stones, especially in developed nations.[33]

In South Carolina, 8 children in 100,000 got kidney stones in 1997. Ten years later in 2007, this increased to 19 children in 100,000. And girls showed higher rates than boys: 21.9 compared to 15.3. In the graphs below (fig. 5), you can see how kidney stone rates increased in Minnesota. The biggest increase was among 15- to 19-year-olds—with an increase of 26% over five years. The risk of kidney stones in childhood has doubled!

Iceland saw an increase in childhood kidney stones and went from 4 children in 100,000 in 1999 to 11 children in 100,000 in 2004. The hardest hit were girls aged 13 to 17, where it rose from 10 in 100,000 to 39 in 100,000. We're not sure why.

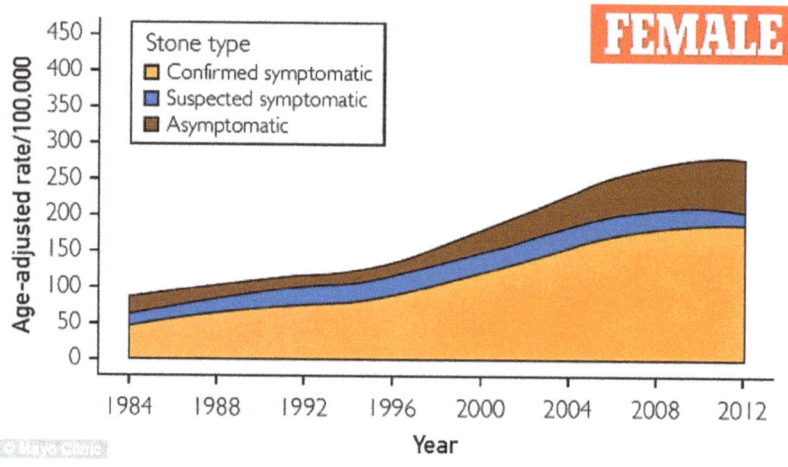

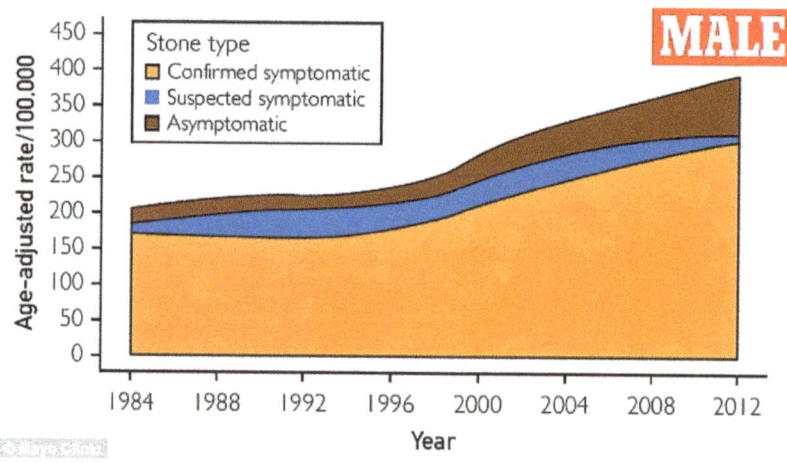

**Figure 5:** *Increase of age-adjusted kidney stone rates. Data from the Mayo Clinic in Rochester, Minnesota, from 1984 to 2012. The increase in females shows this is no longer a predominantly male illness.*

This stone burden comes with a great cost. In 2000, the total cost of caring for patients with kidney stones in the United States was estimated at $2.1 billion USD. This includes $971 million for inpatient, $607 million for outpatient and $490 million for emergency services. From 1994 to 2000, this cost increased 50% with outpatient services increasing to 53% of the total.[34] Due to population growth and the rising prevalence of obesity and diabetes, the cost of caring for kidney stones is estimated to increase by $1.24 billion USD per year by 2030.[35]

## Salt and kidney stones

So, what is the link between salt intake and kidney stones? Well, high salt intake is not the only factor. Some argue that low urinary volumes combined with high salt and protein intake, and low vegetable consumption (what we often see in the typical Western diet) may be responsible for the upsurge in kidney stones.[36] Higher ambient temperatures (air temperature of immediate surroundings) and genetic factors can also play a role.

Salt intake in the United States continues to increase. According to the National Academy of Science, the sodium intake for children 6 to 11 years old in the United States has increased from 200 mg in the 1970s to 3,000 mg in the 2000s.[37] That is right, from two hundred to over three thousand milligrams per day! Nowadays, daily sodium recommendations in the United States for anyone older than age 2 is less than 2,300 mg for healthy individuals and less than 1,500 mg for people considered at risk, for example, those with chronic kidney disease or congestive heart failure. In reality, 88% of Americans consume more than 2,300 mg of salt each day and 99% consume more than 1,500 mg each day.[38] The average daily consumption of sodium in children over 2 years old is 3,266 mg; for 12- to 19-year-olds, it's 3,310 mg. Unfortunately, 65% of that sodium comes from food purchased in stores and 25% comes from restaurant food.[39]

Efforts directed at the processed-food industry, large national restaurant chains and organizations to lower the salt in their products have been in vain in the United States.

Canadian data reveals a similar pattern. One study reported an average sodium intake of 2,388 mg for children age 1 to 8; 3,412 mg for youths age 9 to 18; 3,587 mg for males age 19 and older; and 2,684 for females age 19 and older.[40] These numbers are almost identical to the US data. While this data is based on dietary surveys and may not be accurate, we can estimate salt consumption from the amount of urinary sodium excreted per day, which averages 158 millimoles (mmol) per day, or 3,641 mg per day.[41] This was validated in multiple countries.

## How does high salt intake cause kidney stones?

So, how does our daily salt consumption cause kidney stones? It works this way: The more sodium you eat or drink, the more sodium the kidneys must remove.[42] The more sodium your kidneys have to get rid of, the more calcium gets wasted (fig. 6). There's a close relationship between sodium and calcium. For every 100 mmol (2,300 mg) of urinary sodium you excrete, your urinary calcium increases by 1 mmol (40 mg).[43] This is seen in adolescents as well.[44] The more calcium the kidneys waste, the more calcium becomes available for rapid formation of crystals in the urine. Some calcium salts, such as calcium oxalate, can't be dissolved and form crystals which eventually can form stones. Salt intake may be the single most important reason for the worldwide increase of kidney stones across all ages, particularly in children and adolescents.

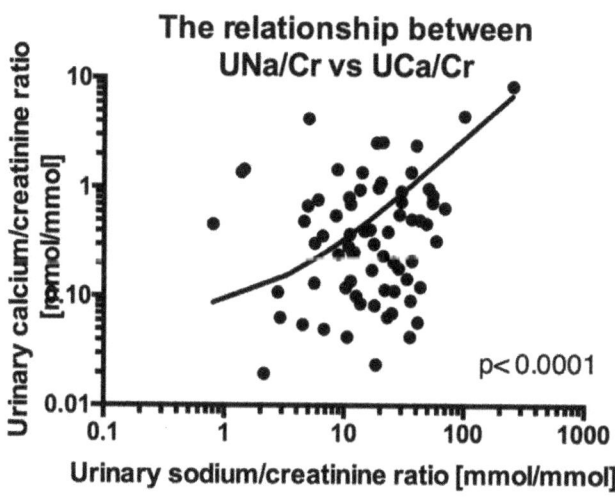

**Figure 6:** *The relationship between urinary calcium excretion (x-axis) and urinary sodium excretion (y-axis). The higher the urinary sodium/creatinine ratio is, the higher the urinary calcium/creatinine ratio.*

## The benefits of high potassium intake

You may be wondering if salt replacements such as potassium salts are a healthier alternative. Indeed, potassium is helpful in most people, *unless* you have advanced chronic kidney disease. Higher urinary potassium decreases the amount of calcium excreted in the urine.[45] The more potassium you eat, the more calcium your kidneys can reabsorb, which reduces calcium wasting.

Potassium-rich foods include avocados, bananas, oranges, cantaloupe, apricots (dried or fresh), grapefruit, prunes, raisins, dates, cooked spinach, cooked broccoli, potatoes, sweet potatoes, peas, cucumbers, zucchini, eggplant, pumpkins, acorn squash, salmon and legumes such as lima beans, pinto beans, kidney beans, white beans, soybeans and lentils. Certain juices such as orange juice, tomato juice (although there often is a lot of added salt), prune juice, apricot juice and grapefruit juice are also excellent sources of potassium. Just be careful if you have chronic kidney disease. With low kidney function, potassium levels may increase in your blood. It may not be safe to eat a high-potassium diet.

High intake of potassium also contributes to more citrate in the urine, and citrate inhibits crystal formation. When you have low levels of urinary citrate, the risk of developing kidney stones increases.[46] Citrate is a weak organic acid that's found in food; it enters your body mainly through diet. Citric acid exists in a variety of fruits and vegetables, most notably citrus fruits. Lemons and limes have particularly high concentrations of the acid. Studies show that 10 millilitres (mL) (or two teaspoons) of lemon juice concentrate taken three times a day can help reduce the risk of new kidney stone formation. Foods that are high in citrate are also high in potassium.

High potassium foods also provide benefits to blood sugar levels, blood pressure levels, and heart and kidney health (unless you already have chronic kidney disease, in which case your kidneys can no longer remove excess potassium and it may stay in your body); aid the digestive process; help keep the body well moisturized; reduce the possibility of bone-structure problems, especially osteoporosis; boost energy levels; are good for the brain and nervous system; and contribute to mental well-being. Consuming a lot of potassium can diminish the impact of a high-salt diet and reduce calcium in the urine towards normal values.[47]

Kidney stones can occur for reasons other than diet:
- Genetic diseases such as cystinuria
- High uric acid excretion, possibly due to consuming a lot of high-fructose corn starch syrup, which gets converted to uric acid in the urine
- Hyperoxaluria
- Other conditions

Some of these are not preventable. However, lowering salt intake appears to be the easiest and simplest way to dramatically improve health and reduce the dependence on health care.

## Summary

Kidney stones are increasing, and the formerly "adult disease" is becoming a disease in children. This condition is chronic and may be associated with a lower life expectancy. Passing kidney stones may be the most painful health issue known to humans. The sharp increase among teenagers, especially girls, is worrisome. Lowering the salt intake may be the simplest option to reduce kidney stones in all of us.

# Chapter 3:
# High Blood Pressure and Salt

## High blood pressure crisis in a young man

Jeremy was 21 years old. Both his parents were overweight and had limited resources. He mostly ate processed foods. His diet was typically filled with high carbohydrates (sugars) and high sodium. He liked his sweet stuff, such as sugary drinks and sodas. Jeremy also drank three cans of beer a day and preferred hard liquor. He was six feet tall and weighed 280 pounds, with a body mass index (BMI) of 37.9 kg/m². A normal BMI is between 18.5 and 25 kg/m²; a BMI between 25 and 30 kg/m² is considered overweight; and a BMI over 30 kg/m² is obese.

Jeremy's grades in high school were poor so he couldn't get into college. He was working at a fast food place for minimum wage. For about six months, he suffered from terrible headaches. He had trouble concentrating, and his math skills weren't good. He took two to three painkillers a day but didn't see a doctor. He was always tired, sleeping only four hours a night. He spent too much time with bad influences as well and was planning to binge drink on another night out. For a full week, he had nosebleeds every single day. He decided to ride his bike to meet his friends even though it was a very hot and humid summer night. The temperature was 31°C (88°F), with a humidity index of 38°C (100°F). Jeremy hadn't ridden a bicycle in months. After riding only a few hundred metres, he fainted on his bike and crashed into bushes.

When Jeremy woke up, he didn't know where he was—which was in intensive care at the hospital. His head was covered in bandages. A monitor was beeping. It was about midday. Jeremy couldn't feel his right arm or leg. He tried to speak but couldn't make any sound. His headache was so severe each thought added more pain. When Jeremy came into the hospital, his blood pressure was 240 over 130 mmHg (normal blood pressure is 120 over 80 mmHg). A young nurse told him in a soft voice: "You've had an accident and ended up in the hospital, Jeremy. You had a high blood pressure (hypertensive) crisis and a stroke while riding your bike."

The doctors and nurses gave him treatment for high blood pressure using strong medications. It took five days to slowly lower his dangerously high blood pressure. Based on the imaging, Jeremy had something called posterior reversible encephalopathy syndrome (PRES). They had to repeat the imaging because of the risk he had suffered a small stroke as well. PRES is a syndrome characterized by headaches, confusion, seizures and visual loss. It may occur due to a number of causes but predominantly severe high blood pressure. They did a magnetic resonance imaging MRI of Jeremy's brain and saw areas of swelling. Usually, the symptoms resolve themselves after a period of time, although visual changes sometimes remain. In Jeremy's case, he suffered more than PRES and had a real stroke on the left side of his brain, which affected his right arm and leg.

Both Jeremy's parents suffered from high blood pressure and were taking medication to lower it. Jeremy spent agonizing months in the hospital, followed by rehabilitation. After three months, he regained control of his left arm and hand. However, he still couldn't walk. He is now on three blood pressure medications and was told he may need further medication for the rest of his life. After six months of rehabilitation, he could walk with a walker, but he'll never regain complete function of his right leg.

This is a sad story. It appears that Jeremy may have had undiagnosed high blood pressure for a very long time. Mostly, high blood pressure doesn't give you any symptoms. Jeremy had a lot of warning signs, such as nosebleeds, headaches and difficulty with math. He is recovering, especially as he is now watching his diet and has had incredible success with weight loss. Jeremy is now 230 pounds and works closely with his dietitian.

## Epidemiology of high blood pressure

Jeremy's story is not uncommon. He has one of the most common chronic illnesses in the Western world: high blood pressure (or hypertension). In his case, there is clearly a genetic predisposition, which was worsened by his obesity and lifestyle choices.

High blood pressure is a long-term "chronic" medical condition in which the blood pressure in the arteries is elevated. High blood pressure alone often doesn't cause symptoms. Long-term high blood pressure, however, is a major risk factor for coronary artery disease, stroke, heart failure, atrial fibrillation (quivering or irregular heartbeat), peripheral vascular disease, vision loss, chronic kidney disease and dementia. This is the reason why high blood pressure is called the "silent killer".

High blood pressure is the most prevalent chronic disease in the United States, as well as in the province of Ontario, Canada. Fifty percent of Ontario residents over the age of 40 suffer from this condition. The annual rate of new cases for the entire Canadian population is about 32 in 1,000 people (ranging between 22.3 to 32.8), which is about the same as for Ontario (31.1).[48] It is three times more prevalent than asthma and chronic obstructive pulmonary disease, five times more prevalent than diabetes and ten times more prevalent than stroke. A recent US study of 16,103 participants shows the percentage diagnosed with high blood pressures within different age groups (see Table 3-1).[49]

**Table 3-1:** Comparison of high blood pressure and treatment by age.[49]

| Age group | High blood pressure [%] | Treatment Indicated [%] | Untreated [%] | Treatment goals not met [%] |
|-----------|-------------------------|--------------------------|---------------|------------------------------|
| 20–34 | 17.4 | 6.9 | 67.6 | 58.6 |
| 35–49 | 39.2 | 24.4 | 41.8 | 50.4 |
| 50-64 years | 62.3 | 51.4 | 31.0 | 51.9 |
| over 65 | 77.7 | 77.0 | 27.0 | 63.1 |
| Overall population | 46.8 | 36.9 | 33.2 | 56.7 |

You can see that over age 50, the percentage of people with high blood pressure rises dramatically. You can also see that the vast majority have not been treated adequately. All of these inadequately treated individuals are at risk of developing complications from high blood pressure, such as heart attacks, strokes (like the unfortunate Jeremy) and even death.

Not all high blood pressure is considered the same.[50] A blood pressure like Jeremy's (240 over 130 mmHg) is called a hypertensive crisis.

**Table 3-2:** Blood pressure type measurements for people older than 13 years of age.

| Blood pressure type | Measurement (mmHg) |
|---------------------|---------------------|
| Normal blood pressure | 120/80 |
| Elevated blood pressure | 120–129/80 |
| High blood pressure | > 130/80 |
| Stage 1 high blood pressure | 130–139/80–89 |
| Stage 2 high blood pressure | 140+/90 |
| Hypertensive crisis | 180+/120+ |

In children, the definition of high blood pressure is more complicated. The blood pressure of a newborn is about 60/40 mmHg in keeping with previous blood pressure readings, and then it increases with height, until puberty. That means the main factor for determining high blood pressure in children is height.[51]

If you want to find out what is normal for your child, you can download the Ped(z) pediatric calculator or use their online calculator at pedz.de.[52] You can calculate to the 5th, 50th, 90th, 95th and 99th percentiles for blood pressure. This program is free and available for multiple platforms; however, it was developed in Germany and is based on German children, who are taller than North American children. You can change to the AHA, which stands for American Heart Association. You will need your child's height in centimetres, date of birth, and sex.

## How to measure blood pressure

It's important to talk a little bit about how to diagnose high blood pressure. The most frequent blood pressure measurement is called "casual blood pressure". Getting a correct casual blood pressure measurement is key to correctly diagnosing high blood pressure. Blood pressure is most often measured with a device known as a sphygmomanometer (blood pressure monitor), which consists of a stethoscope, arm cuff, dial, pump and valve. You should be comfortably seated and resting for three minutes before your blood pressure is taken. Other electronic devices include oscillometric machines and, in the past, mercury sphygmomanometers; however, there are now concerns about the safety of mercury. If three measurements are done properly at different times, and *all* are above normal, there is a high likelihood that you have high blood pressure. There is only one benign condition, the so-called "white coat high blood pressure". It is a phenomenon in which people have a blood pressure level above the normal range in a clinical setting, though they do not exhibit it in other settings. The diagnosis of white coat high blood pressure is made by ambulatory 24-hour blood pressure monitoring, which involves wearing a device that monitors your blood pressure over 24 hours.[53, 54]

## History of blood pressure measurement

It may be interesting to share a little about the history of blood pressure measurement. The Ancient Egyptians had been indirectly measuring the heartbeat.[55] They conceptualized a heartbeat and circulation, but thought the arteries contained air.[56] Stephan Hales (1677–1761), an English clergyman, was the first to directly measure arterial blood pressure by conducting experiments on horses (fig. 7). He used a fixed glass tube and described how the blood rose in the tube eight feet, three inches, perpendicular to the heart, and when it was at full height, it rose and fell at and after each pulse (two, three or four inches).[57]

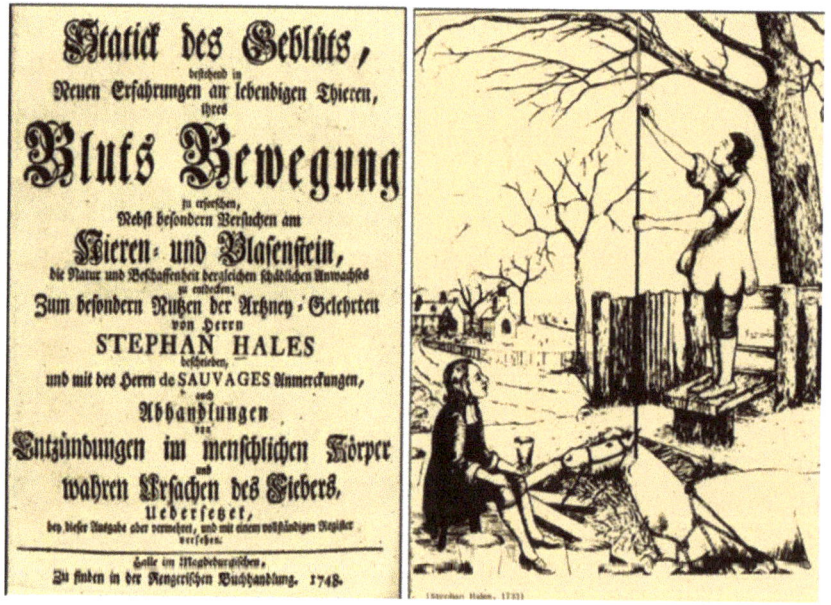

**Figure 7:** *First direct measurement of blood pressure by Stephan Hales.*

This crude and invasive method was later refined. Scientist Étienne-Jules Marey (1830–1904) used counter pressure to overcome the arterial pressure. He improved this device in 1860 by enclosing the arm in a glass chamber filled with water, which was connected to both a sphygmograph (which created a line graph of the pulse) and a kymograph (which traced the record of muscles spasms on a rotating cylinder). Fifteen years later, physician Samuel Siegfried Karl Ritter von Basch (1837–1905) developed a machine that used compression of the artery on the limb; it was the first device to measure blood pressure without cutting into a blood vessel.[58] In 1886, physician Scipione Riva-Rocci (1863–1937) published his landmark paper that prompted the development of the present-day non-invasive easy-to-use cuff-based technique (fig. 8).

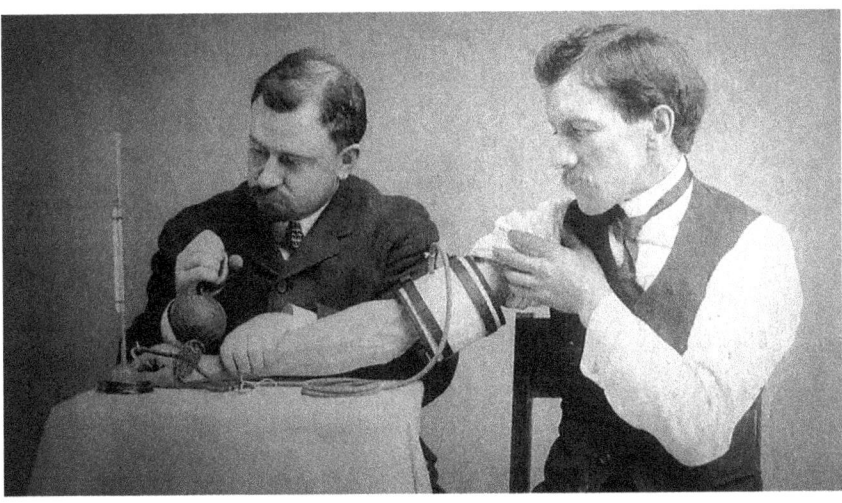

**Figure 8:** *Non-invasive measurement of blood pressure as described by Scipione Riva-Rocci.*

In the United States, the new Riva-Rocci cuff was first introduced into clinical practice at Johns Hopkins Hospital by Cook and Briggs.[59] They did not believe that cuff size influenced the blood pressure reading, so they used a single rubber bladder covered by a canvas case on all their patients, including patients as young as 2 years old. They expanded our understanding of blood pressure by reporting it under various circumstances, such as shock and hemorrhage, and in obstetrics.[60] Although the measurements reported by all three physicians were obtained by palpating the pulse in the arm, Riva-Rocci used a mercury sphygmomanometer in the clinic.[61]

Finally, Russian surgeon Nikolai Korotkoff (1874–1920) described the sounds heard when a stethoscope was placed under the blood pressure cuff over the artery at the elbow.

**Table 3-3:** Korotkoff's five sound phases

| Korotkoff's phase | Description of sound |
|---|---|
| Phase I | Clear tapping tone (systolic blood pressure) |
| Phase II | Tapping softens with a swishing element |
| Phase III | Like phase I, but with distinct sharpening |
| Phase IV | Abrupt muffling of sounds |
| Phase V | All sounds stop (diastolic blood pressure) |

In this process, the bladder was inflated beyond the palpable pulse pressure and then slowly deflated. This became the gold standard and is still used today to measure blood pressure by hand. In this method, the first audible sounds indicate the systolic blood pressure (phase I), which is the upper number. The disappearance of those sounds indicates the diastolic blood pressure (phase V), which is the lower number. In children, we use phase IV, when the sound suddenly becomes a lot softer for the diastolic blood pressure number.[62]

Figure 9 shows a non-invasive blood pressure measurement with an aneroid machine. Aneroid machines require frequent calibrations. Mercury sphygmomanometers are more exact, but these have disappeared in the hospitals because of safety concerns. Today, we often use oscillometric machines. They don't actually measure the systolic blood pressure but rather the arterial pulse, which is when the artery expands because the heart suddenly contracts and increases blood volume in the artery. Systolic and diastolic blood pressure are then calculated using machine-specific algorithms. These machines are quite accurate.

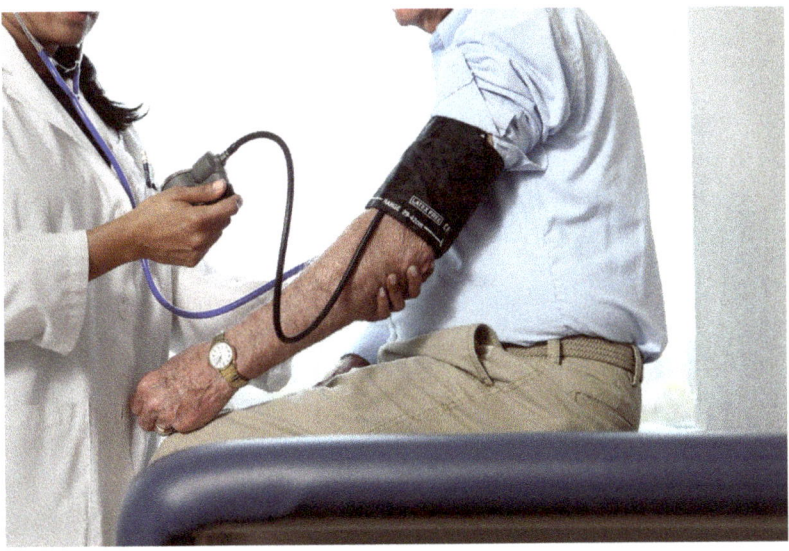

**Figure 9:** *Modern office blood pressure measurement using an aneroid device.*

## What are the causes of high blood pressure?

There are clearly secondary causes of high blood pressure that may be difficult to avoid. These include the following:

- Diseases of the kidney at the kidney filters (1–2%)
- Diseases of the kidney at the kidney vessels (5–34%)
- Primary aldosteronism, a hormonal disorder (8–20%)
- Obstructive sleep apnea (25–50%)
- Drug- or alcohol-induced high blood pressure (2–4%)

Of course, diabetes can also cause high blood pressure. Moreover, there are some rare causes:

- Pheochromocytoma (rare tumour of the adrenal gland tissue)
- Cushing syndrome
- Disorders of the thyroid gland, such as hypothyroidism or hyperthyroidism

- Aortic coarctation (a narrowing of the main vessel coming from the heart, affecting mostly young patients)
- Primary hyperparathyroidism, resulting in high calcium
- Congenital adrenal hyperplasia (a rare hormonal disorder due to two enzyme defects)
- Mineralocorticoid excess syndrome
- Acromegaly

A pediatric nephrologist has to rule out all of these. But the vast majority of high blood pressure in adults is the so-called idiopathic high blood pressure—high blood pressure that doesn't have a known secondary cause, which is also called primary hypertension.

Detailed screening for secondary causes of high blood pressure is not required in adults over age 30 unless it is drug-induced, drug-resistant, abrupt onset, increase of previously controlled high blood pressure, malignant high blood pressure, onset of diastolic high blood pressure in older adults or unprovoked low plasma potassium value. The rest is called primary high blood pressure or essential high blood pressure (which essentially means the health providers do not fully understand the cause). Primary high blood pressure can result from multiple factors, including blood plasma volume and activity of the hormones that regulate blood volume and pressure. It is also influenced by environmental factors such as stress and lack of exercise.

Not only is high blood pressure the number one cause of death and cardiovascular morbidity (rate of disease in a population), it is also the costliest of all cardiovascular diseases. One in three US adults has high blood pressure. Individuals with high blood pressure spend nearly $2,000 USD ($2,618 CAD) more on annual health care than their non-hypertensive peers. A recent US study showed patients with high blood pressure spent $9,089 annually and had $1,920 higher annual adjusted incremental expenses, 2.5 times the inpatient cost, almost double the outpatient cost and nearly triple the prescription medication expenses. Based on the prevalence of high blood pressure in the United States, the hypertensive population's costs are $131 billion USD per year more than the non-hypertensive population.[63]

Assuming that 26% of Ontario citizens have high blood pressure, and looking at the 2019 population of 14,446,515 people, this would amount to a cost of $44.7 billion CAD for Canada's most populous province.

## Salt and high blood pressure

It has long been known that higher salt intake was associated with higher blood pressure; however, we didn't have strong evidence of this until recently. But before examining the evidence, let's look at the reasons why.

Eating salt results in its absorption and an increase in the amount of sodium in your blood stream. Sodium concentration in the blood must be maintained in a very tight, delicate balance. Too much sodium will lead to fluid retention, which increases the circulating blood volume and raises blood pressure. The kidneys must remove the excess sodium and water, which is done through the tubules. This requires a delicate balance of sodium and potassium to pull the water into the collecting channels of the kidneys and subsequently into the bladder. If you eat too much salt and the kidneys can no longer keep up, the extra fluid causes increased blood vessel resistance, which increases blood pressure. Over time, this extra strain can damage the kidneys and you can develop chronic kidney disease. We've found that patients with chronic kidney disease have much higher tissue sodium in their thighs (and other parts) compared to those without kidney disease. This is also the reason why a diuretic (a drug that makes you urinate more often), such as hydro-chlorothiazide, is the most widely used treatment of high blood pressure.[64]

High blood pressure is the most prevalent chronic disease. The typical age of onset used to be 60 years old, but it's gradually decreased to 40 years old. However, older people eat less salt. Then, how can that be? To explain this, you have to look at organ types. We have two types of organs: branching and non-branching. You can repair the non-branching organs such as the liver or the brain until you're 100 years old.[65] By contrast, the branching organs—the pancreas, lungs and kidneys—mature at a certain age and then begin to decline. For example, kidneys have nephrons that act as blood filters. You have about a million nephrons (the maximum amount) at 36 weeks in the womb. Once nephrons are mature, the kidney can start to function. The number of nephrons you have relates to how well your kidneys will function. As you age, your number of nephrons decreases, which means a slow loss of the kidney filters, a decline in the rate at which your kidneys filter blood and a decrease in kidney function.[66] In one study of donor kidneys at the Mayo Clinic and Cleveland Clinic, they found the number of viable nephrons declined from roughly 1 million at age 18 to less than 400,000 at age 70.[67] It makes sense then that we become more sensitive to salt as we age; the lower number of nephrons (blood filters) eventually cannot keep up with increased fluid.

The strongest evidence for linking salt intake with high blood pressure comes from multiple clinical trials in an approach called meta-analysis, which combines data from multiple studies. A recent meta-analysis of 34 trials with 3,230 participants showed that modestly reducing salt intake for at least four weeks can make a significant drop in blood pressure without any other intervention, even when differences in age, ethnic group and blood pressure status were accounted for. The study supports the fact that the more you reduce your sodium intake, the more your blood pressure will fall. Reducing salt intake will lower blood pressure and reduce the risk for cardiovascular disease.[68]

## Salt and health care costs

How do these changes relate to health care costs? We can learn a lot from the Finnish salt laws. Finland started a successful salt reduction campaign in 1970, in North Karelia. Reducing salt intake became a nation-wide campaign in 1986 and salt-labelling legislation was put into effect June 1, 1993. Salt labelling regulations were applied to all food items, and foods high in salt had to be labelled with a "high salt content" warning. This means the label must be present if the salt content is more than 1.3% in bread, 1.8% in sausages, 1.4% in cheese, 2.0% in butter and 1.7% in breakfast cereals or crisp bread. This warning label has been very effective and has led to markedly reduced average salt content in most of the important food categories. The government also worked with the food industry to lower the sodium content by using a variety of substitutes, such as low sodium and high potassium, calcium or magnesium salts.[69] Finland has subsequently seen a 40% drop in average sodium intake, a drop in average blood pressure levels and an 80% drop in deaths due to stroke.[70] Strategies like the ones in Finland (reformulation, food labelling and media campaigns) are more effective than individually focused interventions.[71]

If we can push the average age of the onset of high blood pressure back to age 60, rather than the current age of 40, by adopting similar measures, this would mean an average saving of health care costs of about $11,900 CAD per person per year for 20 years or about $287,000 per person. When we look at Ontario again, with 26% of Ontario citizens having high blood pressure, this would amount to $17.9 trillion over 20 years for Canada's most populous province. (This is calculated assuming that there's no inflation.) Is that not enough motivation for simply copying what Finland started four decades ago?

## Summary

Overall, the link between high blood pressure and salt intake is well established. The example of Finland shows that disease and deaths due to high blood pressure can be reduced substantially by reducing salt intake by 40%. This is profound! This saves almost a quarter of a million dollars per person over 20 years. In Canada's smaller cities, you can still get a house for that amount of money. The health care savings from adoption of the Finnish salt laws could help ease the deficit of the Ontario government. It's unclear why we're almost 40 years behind Finland.

# Chapter 4:
# Osteoporosis and Salt

## Horrible outcome for a 60-year-old lady

Linda had five children and three grandchildren. She breastfed all of her children for more than a year. Linda broke her hip when she delivered her last child. A few years back, when attempting to lift her granddaughter, she fractured her spine. She was told that she had osteoporosis (bone loss) and that was the reason for her constant back pain. A couple years ago, she was tying her shoelaces and felt a crushing pain in her back again. After visiting the emergency room, she learned that she had suffered another compression fracture of one of her vertebrae.

At age 60, Linda could not walk for much more than a couple hundred yards without pain. Her back was round, and she had quite a belly. She drank two to three pints of beer every day and was also a heavy smoker. Her household income was low, and most of the food she ate was processed and from cheap sources. She had taken a prescription drug called alendronate for several years. She was also seeing a specialist who asked her to consume a high-calcium diet and sufficient protein.

Linda didn't really like dairy foods as they made her sick (she was lactose intolerant). She was told to take vitamin D but that wasn't covered by insurance. She was also told to eat bok choy, kale, mustard greens and broccoli, all of which she hated. She was told not to lie down after taking her medicine because it could get stuck in her food pipe and to take it first thing in the morning. Linda always felt nauseated from the medication. She constantly suffered from heartburn and had been diagnosed with an ulcer twice. Extra-strength ibuprofen was not helping, and she took a lot of it. She was also told there was a concern with her kidney function and she might have to stop taking the alendronate. Her doctor recommended menopausal hormone therapy, but she didn't want it—her hot flashes had finally stopped. More recently, as she was renewing her driver's licence, she became concerned about the curve in her back, her sloping shoulders and her hunched posture as she'd shrunk 2.5 inches.

Not that long ago, in the morning when Linda was pushing herself up from bed, her right leg suddenly snapped—like a cracked mug breaking on a whim. She was taken to the hospital and told that she had broken her femur. The orthopaedic doctor said that normal bones don't just break like that. After imaging, he explained that she had suffered a lot of microfractures; her femur was like a honeycomb that had gradually become more fragile and gotten squashed from too great a force. It was an atypical fracture; her bone was crumblier than expected. Linda received an artificial hip because the surgeon was concerned she would get femoral neck shortening (fig. 10).

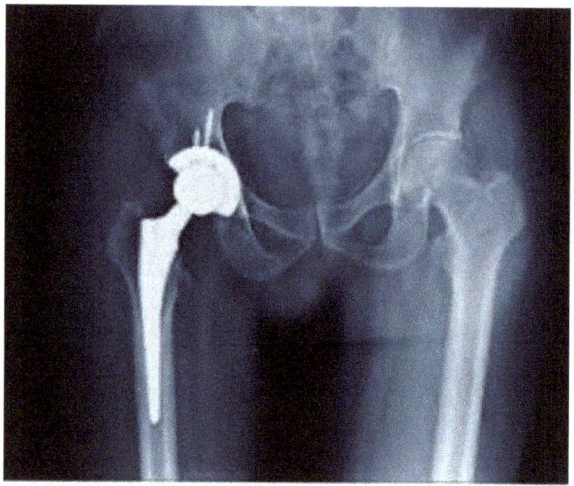

shutterstock.com • 459856552

**Figure 10:** *Artificial hip shown on X-ray.*

While the surgery went well, Linda later experienced a catastrophic failure. At first, she suffered a screw fracture, and then she needed a total hip replacement. A couple years later, the cobalt-chrome femoral head eroded through the socket of her artificial hip. She was found to have metal debris and a large fluid collection in her thigh. This had become infected, and she later died in hospital from the consequences of the overwhelming infection.

## How common is osteoporosis?

Linda had a terrible case of osteoporosis that eventually caused her premature death. You would think that osteoporosis is a disease of older folks, but recently younger and younger patients are being affected by it. In Germany, a country with three times the population of Canada, a person breaks a femur, arm or vertebral body every minute. In that country, six million people over the age of 60 have severe osteoporosis.[72] Recently, we've found this disease is claiming younger and younger patients, and the number of those suffering from the disease is estimated at over 200 million.[73] This number is probably a substantial underestimate.

Approximately 30% of all postmenopausal women in Europe and the United States have osteoporosis (fig. 11). At least 40% of the women and 15–30% of men with osteoporosis will have pathological fractures (broken bones caused by disease, not an injury) in their lifetime.[74, 75] More recent US data suggests that this number is now much higher—in 2010, an estimated 53.6 million.[76] Furthermore, the rate of death within seven days of admission for an osteoporosis-induced hip fracture is 1.3% for the province of Manitoba and 2.0% in New York. This is similar to Linda's poor story. This disease is truly an important public health concern.

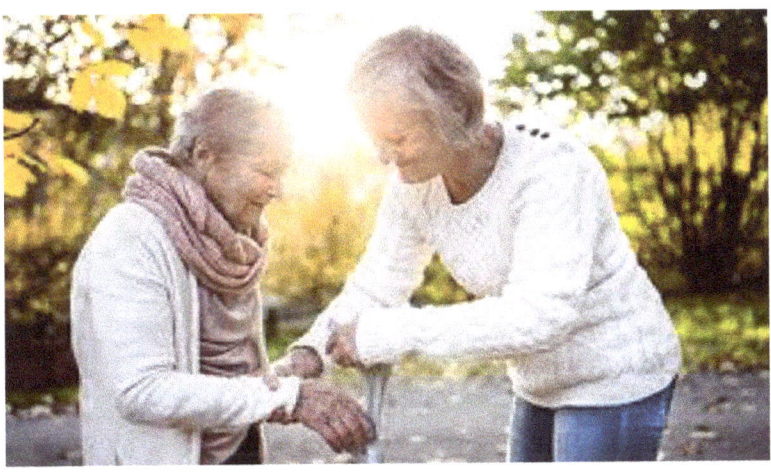

**Figure 11:** *Patient with severe osteoporosis.*

## What is osteoporosis?

Osteoporosis is a disease in which bone is weakened, increasing the risk of fracture (fig. 12). Normally, the bone looks like a honeycomb; in the osteoporotic bone, the holes and spaces are much bigger. Essentially, the bone mineral density is lower than normal. Osteoporosis may be due to lower-than-normal maximum bone mass or greater-than-normal bone loss.

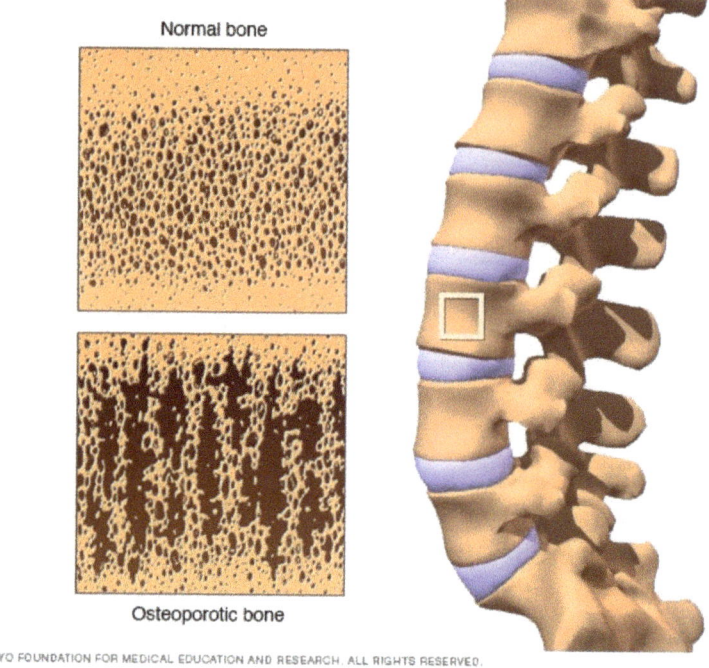

Normal bone

Osteoporotic bone

**Figure 12:** *Normal bone and osteoporotic bone.*

Your bone strength changes throughout your life. Bone mass is a measure of the amount of minerals in your bone; it increases rapidly in childhood, especially during teenage years, and may continue growing until the early twenties. Males have higher bone mass than females. Females achieve their peak bone mass earlier because they finish puberty earlier. Usually around the early twenties, bone is remodelled (mature bone breaking down and new bone forming) and lost at a steady rate for the rest of one's life, for both males and females (fig. 13). This is mostly due to loss of the trabecular bone—the spongy, honeycomb-like inner layer of the bone. Eventually, some people develop so much bone loss that the remaining bone fails structurally from stresses and fractures that arise from doing ordinary physical activity—such as when Linda pushed herself out of bed.

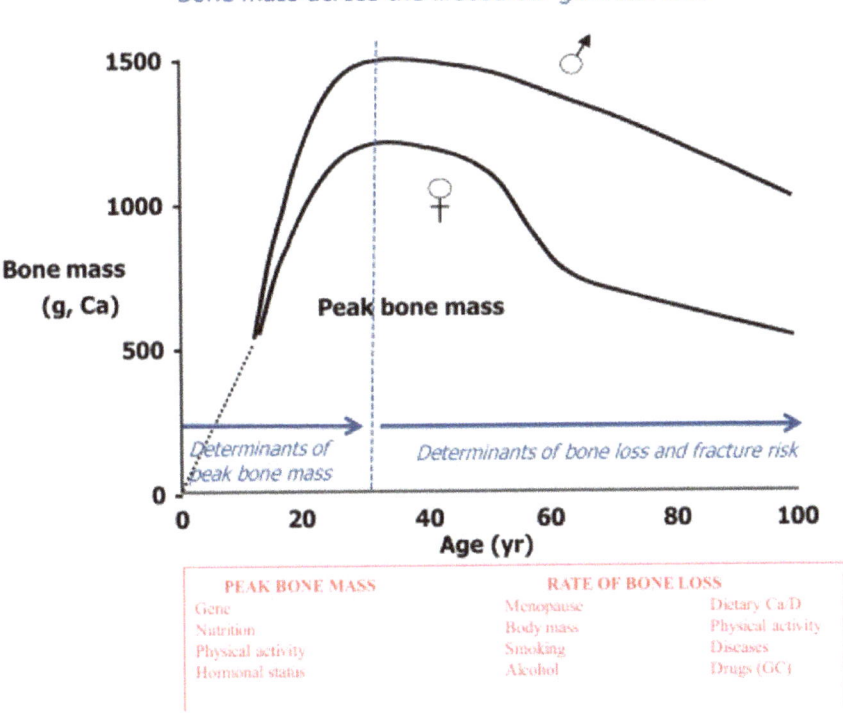

**Figure 13:** *Bone mass over the course of a life.*

Peak bone mass is decreasing because of nutrition, and there are a number of reasons why. Our sedentary lifestyle contributes to a decrease of peak bone mass. The widespread use of oral contraceptives in adolescence seems to interfere with bone mineral mass development.[77] The biggest nutritional factor, however, is salt-induced calcium wasting.

## The cost of osteoporosis

Osteoporosis-associated fractures come with a substantial cost. In a recent Canadian study,[78] the acute care cost (emergency and surgery) for a hip fracture totalled $4,070 per person, with another $19,760 for an average 14-day stay in the hospital. Inpatient medical visits totalled $229. Acute rehabilitation totalled $24,639, and long-term care totalled $74,646. Vertebral fractures were a bit cheaper. On average, every new osteoporosis-associated fracture cost $50,000.

Eighty percent of fractures are caused by osteoporosis.[79] In a Canadian 2007 study, the cost for acute care for hip fractures totalled $619.3 million, and all other fractures cost $552.3 million,[80] with a sum of $1.2 billion. Eighty percent of this is $937.3 million.[81] The cost of osteoporosis is high.

## What causes osteoporosis?

Osteoporosis does not have a single cause. Lifestyle choices, such as diet and exercise, and biological factors can all lead to osteoporosis. The leading cause of osteoporosis is a lack of certain hormones, particularly estrogen in women and androgen in men. Diet has a generous impact on the quality of your bones. Some foods assist bones to remain in good physical condition, while others do not. Calcium and vitamin D are essential nutritional factors for bone growth and maintenance. Other vitamins and minerals such as vitamin B and magnesium support bone health. Protein, caffeine and sodium, if taken in large quantities, can be harmful for bones. Caffeine can lead to calcium loss through the urine. Excessive alcohol use definitely contributes to the development of osteoporosis, as does smoking.

Alcohol has a negative effect on bone health for several reasons.[82] In women, chronic alcohol use can trigger irregular menstrual cycles, a factor that reduces estrogen levels, which increases the risk for osteoporosis. Also, cortisol levels may be elevated in people with alcoholism. Research shows that chronic heavy alcohol use, especially during adolescence and young adult years, can dramatically affect bone health and increase the risk of osteoporosis later in life.[83] When you drink too much (defined as more than two to three ounces of alcohol every day), the result is a decrease in the calcium dissolved in your stomach and absorbed through the lining of the small intestine into your blood stream. Alcohol also interferes with the absorption of vitamin D and calcium by acting on the pancreas. Furthermore, alcohol can damage osteoblasts, the cells that form new bones. This results in abnormal bone remodelling of the skeleton.[84] There is evidence that moderate to severe alcohol intake in postmenopausal women causes lower biochemical markers of bone turnover (products released during the process of bone resorption and replacement).[85]

Smoking is also bad for your bone health. It negatively affects the parathyroid hormone, which regulates calcium levels; reduces levels of vitamin D; reduces estrogen levels; and accelerates bone loss (especially in the femur).[86] Smoking early in life is particularly bad as it reduces your peak bone mass—at the end of adolescence, when your greatest bone mass and strength is achieved—and the more you smoke, the worse the effect is.[87] This has been shown in both young men and women.[88] Adolescent men who started to smoke in puberty have considerably smaller increases in bone mineral content compared to non-smoking adolescent men.

However, the biggest problem for bone health may well be the tsunami of problems rolling towards us because of calcium wasting in the kidneys due to salt. It's been shown that 50% of adolescents with kidney stones already have osteoporosis.

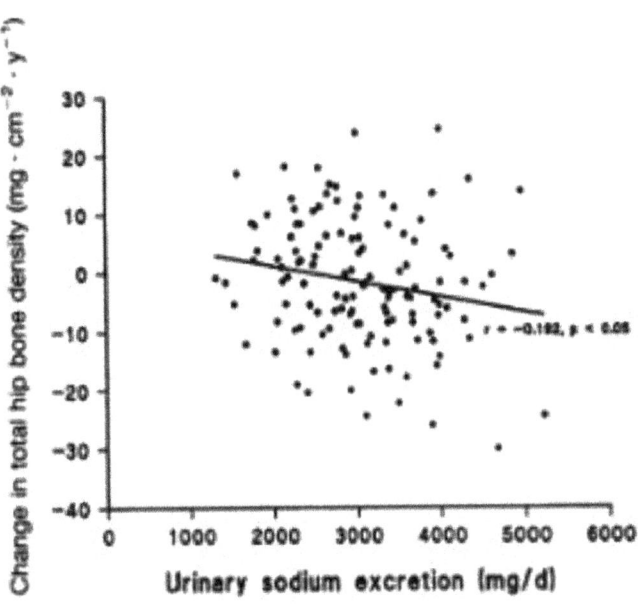

**Figure 14:** *The relationship between urinary sodium excretion per day and change in total hip bone density.*

In a meta-analysis of 39,065 people, the risk of osteoporosis increased in parallel with their salt intake.[89] Unfortunately, there aren't a lot of good studies on osteoporosis in adolescents. There may also be racial differences, as one study has clearly shown that Caucasian girls are at a greater risk of wasting calcium compared to African-American girls.[90] This may be only an issue in adolescents, as the findings could not be replicated in adults.[91, 92]

Osteoporosis is not only a major public health issue, it is also associated with greater risk of disease and even death. In Finland, the 40% reduction in daily sodium intake over the past two decades has resulted in a continuously declining incidence of hip fractures (fig. 15).[93] This compares to the rest of Europe (except Norway), where the incidence has been going up.[94]

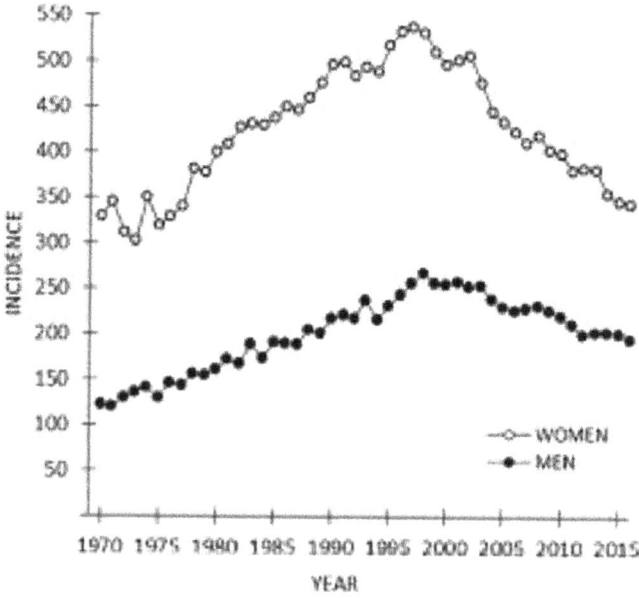

**Figure 15:** *The development of hip fracture incidence rates from 1970 to 2015 in Finland.*

## Summary

The annual cost of osteoporosis-associated fractures in Canada is substantial. If we could adopt the Finnish salt laws and achieve a similar 50% decline of osteoporosis-associated fractures (rather than the meagre 1.2% decrease observed in Canada), we could save about $468.6 million per year. This would also substantially improve longevity and quality of life. Enhancing our current efforts to reduce salt intake in North America will not only bring us better health, it will provide sumptuous savings in health care costs.

# Chapter 5:
# Obesity and Salt

## Catastrophic outcome of morbid obesity

John was 35 years old when his cardiologist told him he had stage 4 heart failure. He had constant and severe debilitating symptoms, even while at rest. His legs were swollen. He felt extremely bloated and had constant shortness of breath, nausea and chest pain. He also suffered from incredible fatigue, even when he woke up in the morning. He had to monitor his weight, and even though he hardly ate at all (because of nausea), he was gaining weight. His doctor told him it was water and further increased the water pills John was taking. His chest X-ray showed a large heart and excess fluid in and around the lungs (fig. 16).

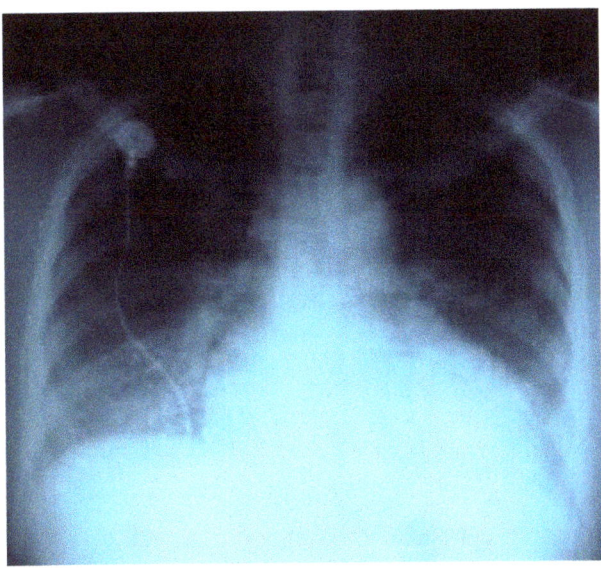

**Figure 16:** *Congestive heart failure image, similar to what John's chest X-ray looks like.*

John was on a lot of medications. These included blood pressure medicines, several water pills, low-dose digitalis (to strengthen his failing heart), antidepressants and opioids. He also needed continuous oxygen. He was told that his heart had a very low function and could no longer pump the blood needed for his huge body. His doctor suggested sacubitril in combination with a blood pressure medicine, and they were waiting for approval. John had been told for years to change his diet and do more exercise, but how? He was unemployed and lived on welfare; his wife bought food on a limited budget. John was on a waiting list for a heart transplant, but his cardiologist said he might not make it while waiting for an organ to become available.

So, what was left for John? He liked his salty food; his favourite was a hamburger with extra bacon and cheese. He had been obese since childhood. His parents (both dead) had been obese as well. John said, "It runs in the family." He always had a craving for salty food. Yes, it made him extra thirsty, and he could easily drink two to three litres of *soda* every day. At age 14, he was the largest and tallest in his class, and he already weighed 300 pounds.

John did not make it to his heart transplant. His cardiologist stated that his heart failed because of high blood pressure and morbid obesity, and because

John ate too much salt. The doctor suspects that bad dietary habits—and possibly even just the high-salt intake—had caused childhood onset obesity, which eventually resulted in heart failure and death.

## Obesity and the role of salt

So, how are salt and obesity linked? There has always been obesity, even before the significant increase of salt intake in the 1980s. However, since the 1980s, obesity rates have been increasing at an alarming rate. The obesity trend in the United States coincides with the introduction of high-fructose corn syrup (as a replacement for sugar) and the massive increase in salt intake in our population (fig. 17 and 18). High-fructose corn syrup was used from the 1970s as a sugar replacement because it was similar to sugar and cheaper to manufacture.

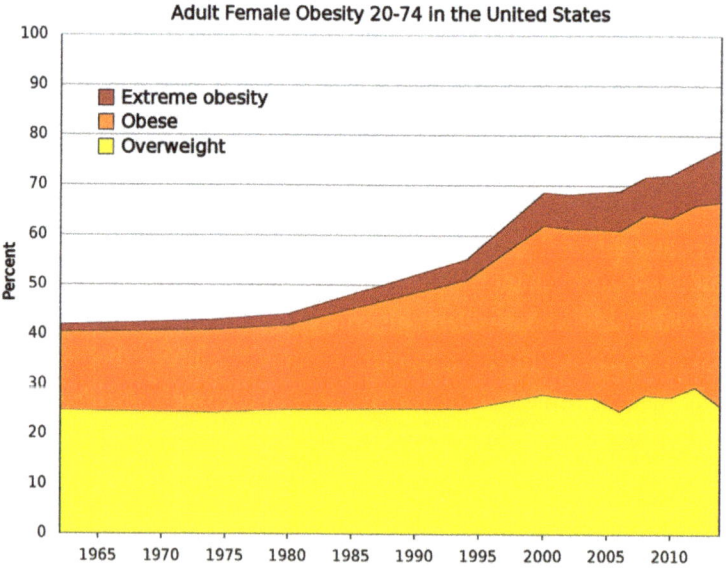

**Figure 17:** *Adult female obesity rates of women aged 20–74.*

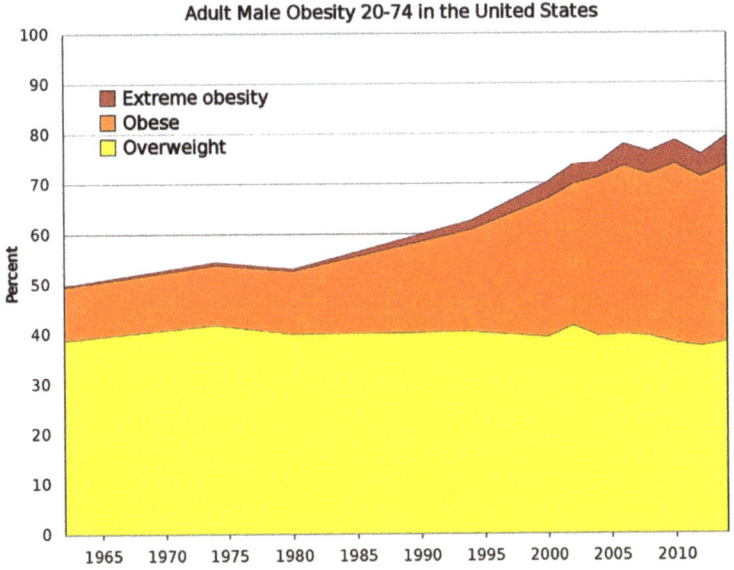

**Figure 18:** *Adult male obesity rates of women aged 20–74*

## Obesity and the food industry

There is a lot of confusion about what's causing the worldwide obesity epidemic. Obesity is caused by a number of factors. In the 1970s, it was proposed that eating too much saturated fatty acids caused coronary artery disease (a disease in which the coronary arteries—the major blood vessels that supply your heart with blood, oxygen and nutrients—are not functioning normally). Cholesterol-containing deposits (plaque) in the arteries and inflammation are usually to blame for coronary artery disease. When plaque builds up, it narrows the coronary arteries, decreasing blood flow to the heart. Eventually, the decreased blood flow may cause chest pain (angina) and shortness of breath. A complete blockage can cause a heart attack.

This is all based on the Framingham Heart Study, a long-term, ongoing cardiovascular study of residents of the city of Framingham, Massachusetts. The study began in 1948 with 5,209 adults and is now on the fourth generation of participants. The study measures the number of cases of high blood pressure and cardiovascular disease and has resulted in more than 1,000 publications.[95] Before this study, we thought higher blood pressure, atherosclerosis (plaque build-up inside your arteries) and higher cholesterol in the blood were part of normal aging. Now we know that cardiovascular health can be influenced by lifestyle and genetic factors.

The study made other major discoveries. It showed that cigarette smoking, obesity, elevated blood pressure and increased cholesterol increase the risk of heart disease.[96] It was discovered that elevated blood pressure increases the risk of strokes. In the 1980s, the study demonstrated that higher HDL (good cholesterol) levels are associated with lower cardiovascular risk. More recently, it was shown that blood pressure that is closer to the higher range (previously labelled "pre-high blood pressure" and now simply called "elevated blood pressure") increases the risk of cardiovascular disease.[97]

Based on the differences of cardiovascular disease between Americans and Europeans, and its association with saturated fat intake, a whole industry has developed. Despite the fact that "association" does not mean cause and effect are related, the food industry replaced the addictive fat in processed food with even more addictive sugars. The industry developed junk food designed to be cheap, long lasting on the shelf and delicious—it became irresistible.

The consumption of very tasty foods and larger portion sizes has resulted in overeating. Most processed foods do not resemble whole foods at all and are designed to get people addicted. By combining food addiction, aggressive marketing and prices that are cheaper than whole foods, the food industry created a perfect storm for an obesity epidemic. Add to that low access to recreation opportunities and high availability of fast food outlets, and you have an environment that is conducive to obesity. There are many convenience stores in areas of the lowest socioeconomic status, where the obesity rates are the highest.[98]

In the poorest area of London, Ontario, for example, there is only one (very expensive) grocery store but a high density of fast food outlets and convenience stores. A study showed that 65% of adolescents in London get their food from convenience stores and fast food outlets. The study concluded that we need large-scale solutions: "Macro-level regulations and policies are required to amend the health-detracting neighbourhood food environment surrounding children and youths' home and school."[99] As obesity often starts during childhood and adolescence, we really need to focus more on the environment we're building.

## High-fructose corn syrup

Among the sugars, high-fructose corn syrup is the worst. High-fructose corn syrup was introduced as a cheaper alternative to cane sugar and beet sugar. High-fructose corn syrup was first marketed in the early 1970s by the Clinton Corn Processing Company (in Clinton, Iowa) using technology licensed from the Japanese Agency of Industrial Science and Technology, where the enzyme was discovered in 1965. To make high-fructose corn syrup, the corn syrup is processed by the enzyme glucose isomerase to convert some of its glucose into fructose. The US Food and Drug Administration has determined that high-fructose corn syrup is a safe ingredient for food and beverage manufacturing.[100]

So, is high-fructose corn syrup worse than regular sugar? Table sugar is made up of both fructose and glucose. What is the difference between fructose and glucose? Fructose is sweeter than glucose and most often added to processed food. To create high-fructose corn syrup, enzymes are added to corn starch to turn the glucose into fructose. Both are simple sugars, but the body processes them differently. Glucose is essential for brain metabolism (converting food into energy). It's metabolized by other organs as well: liver, muscles and fat tissue. It affects blood sugar and insulin levels.

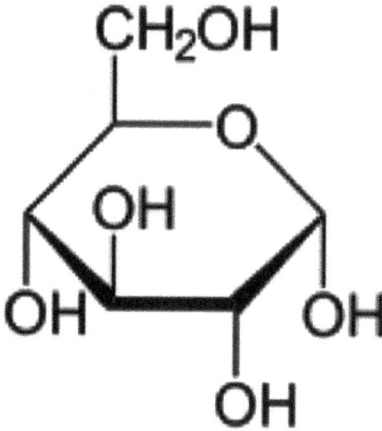

**Figure 19:** *The chemical structure of glucose consists of six carbon atoms in a ring (hexose) and is the most abundant monosaccharide. Most of it comes to the body through food, but it can also be synthesized in the body. It's an essential nutrient for the brain.*

Fructose, by contrast, is a fruit sugar that's primarily metabolized by the liver. Consuming too much fructose may contribute to insulin resistance, obesity, higher LDL (bad) cholesterol and triglycerides. This can lead to metabolic syndrome—a cluster of conditions including abnormalities such as increased blood pressure, high blood sugar and abnormal cholesterol that increase the risk of cardiovascular disease and Type 2 diabetes.[101, 102]

Fructose is not metabolized well in the body. While glucose can be used for almost any cell in the body, fructose must be metabolized in the liver. And there is no limit to how much it will metabolize; the more fructose you eat, the more it's broken down in the liver. It can result in a fatty liver and insulin resistance. The process of breaking down fructose is complex, and its metabolism creates triglycerides, uric acid and free radicals, which are a problem. Triglycerides can damage the liver and build up plaque in the walls of the arteries. Uric acid inhibits production of nitric acid (which helps protect arterial walls). Free radicals can damage cells, enzymes and genes.[103]

In an excellent review in *Diabetes, Metabollic Syndrome and Obesity: Targets and Therapy* journal, Brandon Mai and Liang-Jun Yan state:

The increased consumption of fructose in the average diet through sweeteners such as high-fructose corn syrup (HFCS) and sucrose has resulted in negative outcomes in society through producing a considerable economic and medical burden on our health care system. Ingestion of fructose chronically has contributed to multiple health consequences, such as insulin resistance, obesity, liver disorders and diabetes. Fructose metabolism starts with fructose phosphorylation by fructose kinase in the liver, and this process is not feedback regulated. Therefore, ingestion of high fructose can deplete ATP [or energy], increase uric acid production and increase nucleotide turnover. This review focuses the discussion on the hepatic manifestations of high fructose–implicated liver metabolic disorders such as insulin resistance, obesity due to enhanced lipogenesis, non-alcoholic fatty liver disease (NAFLD), non-alcoholic steatohepatitis (NASH) and type 2 diabetes.[104]

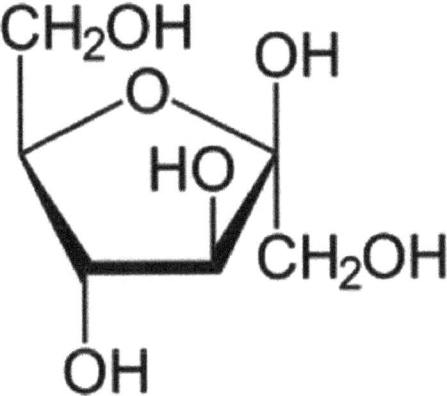

**Figure 20:** *The chemical structure of fructose. Fructose is a pentose, with only five carbon atoms. In high-fructose corn syrup, it is essentially the only monosaccharide component of a large polysaccharide. The European Food Safety Authority has warned: "High intakes of fructose may lead to metabolic complications such as dyslipidaemia, insulin resistance and increased visceral adiposity."*

Not only does fructose go directly into the fat storage cells, in most cases it also causes high uric acid levels. When your body breaks down fructose, purines are released and as these chemical compounds are broken down, uric acid is produced. Uric acid can form painful crystals in the joints, causing gout. Once consumed, fructose can generate uric acid within minutes. A study on fructose-rich beverages and risk of gout in women found that women who drank one can of sugary soda a day had a 74% higher risk of developing gout than women who rarely drank sugary soda. This was based on a study of 78,906 women who were followed over 22 years.[105]

The cost difference between high-fructose corn syrup and beet sugar was a major driver in the use of fructose. But recently, the price has dropped. For example, in December 2017, the cost of high-fructose corn syrup was $0.44 per pound while beet sugar was only $0.35 per pound.[106] Let's hope the food industry will revert to regular sugar so that only half of the carbohydrates go right into our fat storage cells.

## Insulin resistance

Insulin resistance and leptin resistance also contribute to obesity. Insulin is a very important hormone that regulates energy storage, among other things. One of its functions is to get fat cells to store fat and hold onto the fat they already carry. The Western diet promotes the development of insulin resistance.[107] To reduce insulin levels, you must decrease your intake of refined sugar and increase your intake of fibre. Leptin is a hormone that's produced by fat cells; it acts on receptors in the brain to regulate energy balance and body weight. In most cases, obese individuals are not leptin-deficient but rather have high levels of circulating leptin that fail to control body weight regulation. Leptin tells your brain to use its fat stores for energy; when cells in the brain stop recognizing leptin's signals, leptin resistance is occurring. Leptin resistance can also impair other functions, such as lipid and carbohydrate metabolism and the absorption of nutrients in the intestines.[108]

## Mechanisms of high-salt intake causing obesity

There are essentially five ways that consuming a lot of salt leads to obesity:

- It affects the gut flora (microbes).
- It may cause your body to retain more water.
- It produces a progressive increase in thirst; as most people drink sugary beverages rather than water, they are also increasing their fructose intake.
- A diet high in salt usually includes overconsumption of fatty foods.
- It may lead to significant changes in hormones that control our appetite and may have a direct effect on making new fat cells.

On a more scientific level, the following occurs:

1. A high-salt diet activates processes that result in endogenous fructose production—this means we produce the fructose ourselves in our body—and the fructose is then metabolized.[109] A high-salt diet activates the polyol pathway (or sorbitol-aldose reductase pathway) in the liver. First glucose is reduced into sorbitol, and then sorbitol is oxidized into fructose. This further induces leptin resistance and the development of metabolic syndrome and a fatty liver. We are not only eating too much fructose; we are also starting to produce this ourselves owing to a high-salt diet.

2. High-salt intake alters gut flora and increases concentration of plasma trimethylamine N-oxide, which is a metabolite derived from gut bacteria. Trimethylamine N-oxide is an established biomarker (a biological sign) of cardiovascular disease.[110] It may be that a high-salt diet promotes the growth of bacteria that produce toxins that affect the cardiovascular system. It's well established that there is a linkage between gut flora and the development of obesity.[111] We are still in the infancy of understanding how diet and environmental factors affect the gut microbes and how this affects hormone levels and other factors that may influence obesity.

3. Salt may directly influence the generation of fat cells. A recent study of gene expression showed a significant increase in fat-related genes.[112] Studies in Britain and China show that eating an extra gram of salt each day increased the risk of obesity in children by 28% and adults by 26%.[113]

4. Salt also affects the hunger hormone. Ghrelin is a hormone produced mainly by the stomach, with small amounts also released by the small intestine, pancreas and brain. Ghrelin has numerous functions. It is termed the "hunger hormone" because it stimulates appetite, increases food intake and promotes fat storage.[114] Ghrelin increases when you fast (in line with your increase in hunger). In a study in rural China of 38 non-obese healthy subjects aged 25 to 50, high-salt intake resulted in a significant increase of ghrelin levels while fasting.[115]

There may be many additional factors. Research on the connection between high-salt intake and obesity is only in its infancy and needs to be confirmed in large studies. However, the evidence is mounting that high-salt intake has much more impact on obesity rates than we originally thought.

## Summary

There is growing evidence that high-salt intake affects numerous factors that contribute to obesity. These include the impact on the gut flora and hormone levels and the generation of fat cells. It seems compelling to reduce our salt intake to achieve weight loss. Of course, high-sodium foods such as snacks, chips, fast food, fried foods, processed foods and restaurant meals have all been linked to obesity as well. Remember that one of the primary sources of salt in our diet is bread; there is clear evidence that a reduction of white bread, but not whole grain bread, is associated with lower weight gain. (Whole bread has a different composition and a different effect on body weight and abdominal fat.)[116] Of course, these mechanisms are entangled and interconnected.

It's interesting that the United States, Mexico, New Zealand, Hungary, Australia, the United Kingdom, Canada and Chile have higher obesity rates than Finland.[117] While obesity in adults in the rest of the world is increasing, it has decreased in Finland in parallel with the country's salt reduction.[118] The impact of high-salt intake on gut flora and hormone levels warrants further study.[119] Reducing salt intake is a simple measure that may reduce obesity rates, thereby prolonging life expectancy.

# Chapter 6:
# Chronic Kidney Disease and Salt

## Ali cured himself with intermittent fasting

Ali is a highly successful physician working in a private clinic in Florida. His workload is huge—at least 75 hours a week—and he has almost no time for family or other activities. He is on call often and sleeps irregularly, usually operating all night. There is no time to prepare proper meals, so he used to eat a lot of fast food. His weight crept up, and Ali was shocked to see his stomach start to protrude above his waistline. He had not seen his doctor for a routine check-up in years. At 48 years old, he visited his doctor and was shocked to learn he weighed 240 pounds (at 5 feet, 9 inches in height). Ali's blood pressure was elevated. Blood tests revealed high cholesterol, elevated blood sugar and elevated haemoglobin A1c (a marker of blood sugar control over time), and there was protein in the urine—which is unusual. He was diagnosed with Type 2 diabetes and diabetic-related kidney disease.

Ali's doctor said that the kidneys were being overworked (known as "hyperfiltration"). Treatment with diet and large doses of metformin did not improve his blood sugar control, and he was started on insulin. Ali had to follow a strict schedule and regular meals, which was almost impossible for him given his work. He needed blood pressure medicine to keep it normal, but it didn't decrease the protein in his urine. He also developed signs of diabetic nerve disease and restless legs syndrome, and his feet were not getting good blood flow. He was told that his chronic kidney disease might progress to end-stage kidney failure if he didn't achieve better blood sugar control.

Ali decided to take matters into his own hands. He found a website on intermittent fasting, which is an eating pattern that cycles between periods of fasting and eating.[120] It doesn't specify *which* foods you should eat, but rather *when* you should eat them. It's not a diet in the conventional sense but can be more accurately described as an eating pattern that involves daily 16-hour fasting in 24 hours. The benefits of intermittent fasting have been shown in the research done by Dr. Jason Fung and others.

According to research, when you fast, several things happen to your body on a cellular and even molecular level: The body adjusts hormone levels to make stored body fat more accessible. Cells initiate important repair mechanisms. The levels of human growth hormone increase, as much as five-fold.[121] Insulin sensitivity improves and levels of insulin drop dramatically, which improves how fat storage cells are used in the body.[122] There are also important changes in gene expression that make it easier to repair cells. By eating fewer meals, intermittent fasting can also lead to lower caloric intake. Intermittent fasting makes weight loss easier and results in an increase of the metabolic rate.[123]

Ali realized that his fat tissue caused his insulin resistance and that diet and insulin would control his blood sugar but would not give him a cure. His kidneys were already damaged. When he pictured himself on dialysis, awaiting a kidney transplant with amputated legs and dying on the waiting list while not being able to help his own patients anymore, he realized he needed to take action. He took his intermittent fasting to an extreme, and instead of fasting for 16 hours every day, he decided to have only one meal once a day. He also decided to eat his supper only in the form of food with a low glycaemic index (in other words, foods with carbohydrates that would be very high in fibre without raising the blood sugar much). He chose a diet that was mostly made up of meat and legumes and stopped eating bread and anything sweet. He also decided to avoid any processed food and stopped adding salt to his dinners. Of course, this is against any conventional wisdom. It was an incredible effort to convince his doctor to agree to this plan, but eventually the two men decided to give it a try.

The effects were incredible. Ali's weight came down over one year to 170 pounds. His blood pressure improved to a degree that his family doctor wanted to stop the blood pressure medications; however, since there was kidney involvement, they kept Ali on a small dose of a kidney-protective blood pressure medication. His blood pressure benefited from the salt restriction. He came off all insulin and is now only on one tablet of metformin, and he has a perfect haemoglobin level (HbA1c of 5.2%). There is also no more evidence of diabetic kidney disease or protein in the urine. Ali now has hit a wall at 169 pounds and needs to eat about 2,000 calories with his supper to stop further weight loss. When he cheats and eats three meals, he immediately gains three pounds, and it takes him three days to get back to his 169 pounds. His energy level is boosted, and he looks 10 years younger. He continues to work full time. In fact, he works even more than he used to, as he considers his patients his duty and his work a true privilege. Ali is a changed man.

Obviously, this is an amazing story. Ali has incredible willpower and used powerful habits to make these admirable changes. He told me that everything first happened in his head—he wanted this, and he succeeded. When I asked him about ever returning to a normal diet, he said that he's tried but that he always promptly gains weight. According to Ali, there is no turning back. It's a new life—one where he is able to avoid the progression of kidney disease. I am inspired by Ali's success and have also started intermittent fasting using the 16-hour method. In five months, I have lost 35 pounds. I must admit that this diet almost makes you want to go on a hunt for food, 12 to 14 hours after the last meal, but the results are worth it. It gave me the additional energy to write this book.

## How did the low-salt diet help?

Ali's success has a lot to do with his fasting and weight loss, but the low-sodium diet helped. Let's examine the role of salt and chronic kidney disease. The kidneys play an important role in the balance of fluids and electrolytes in the blood in a very tight range. A high-salt diet will alter the sodium balance. When you eat a high-salt diet, there is excess sodium (and chloride); the kidneys must get rid of that excess salt. We already established that this leads to calcium wasting, resulting in kidney stones and thin bones (osteoporosis). Unfortunately, there is more. A high-salt diet causes an increase in the amount of protein in the kidneys.

The main protein in urine is albumin, which is also the most important protein in blood. Normally, only small amounts of albumin are filtered by the kidneys into the urine, as it will be absorbed by kidney tubules.[124] These tubules fine-tune the urine composition. In healthy individuals, the highest level of urine albumin (known as microalbuminuria) is found among those who eat a high-salt diet.[125, 126] A moderate increase in microalbuminuria is an important marker of diabetes mellitus, high blood pressure for kidney diseases, cardiovascular disease, and in diabetics, kidney damage.[127, 128] This is the most devastating complication of diabetes that leads to kidney failure and premature death.[129] Microalbuminuria is central to clinical practice to monitor and treat diabetic kidney disease.

## Salt and microalbuminuria

How does salt affect the amount of albumin in the urine? In animal experiments, a high-salt diet decreased the nephrons in the kidney by 25%, causing the remaining nephrons to enlarge. In this experiment, blood pressure in the mice was normal, but the tissue looked like that of animals with high blood pressure. These findings suggest that salt alone could be responsible and not the high blood pressure.[130] Other animal experiments also suggest that high salt intake may affect those parts of the kidneys that handle sodium. These include proteins in the foot processes of the cells (called podocytes), which filter the blood and prevent the leaking of albumin. Researchers found the kidney filters were also enlarged and there was less nephrin released. (Nephrin is a protein that holds the foot processes together).[131]

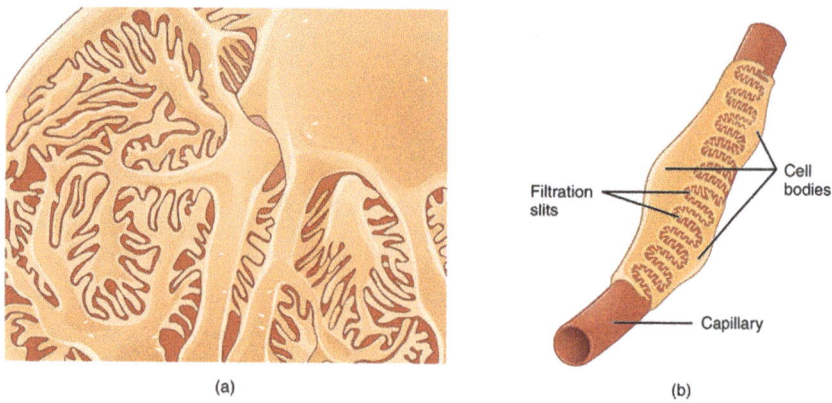

(a)                                              (b)

**Figure 21:** *On the left is a more realistic rendering of how the podocytes ride on top of the capillaries. On the right is a capillary in filtration bodies of the kidneys (called glomeruli) and the principle of how the podocytes interconnect their foot processes. The individual foot processes are connected through a protein called nephrin, which decreases in response to a high-salt diet.*

## Age, salt and kidney-filter size

As mentioned earlier, nephrons (which filter the blood, absorbing what the body needs and excreting the rest into the urine) complete their growth at 36 weeks of gestation.[132] Genetic factors and factors surrounding the environment in the womb affect how many nephrons are created. If the fetal weight is low or the baby is born prematurely, they will not have as many nephrons and this could cause future adult disease, such as high blood pressure, cardiovascular disease, chronic kidney disease and shorter life expectancy.[133, 134] This is known as the Barker hypothesis.[135]

**Table 6-1:** Top 8 countries in 2018 with the greatest number of preterm births[136]

| Country | Number of preterm births |
|---|---|
| India | 3,519,100 |
| China | 1,172,300 |
| Nigeria | 773,600 |
| Pakistan | 748,100 |
| Indonesia | 675,700 |
| United States | 517,400 |
| Bangladesh | 424,100 |
| Philippines | 348,900 |

The WHO website lists some key factors about prematurity:

1. Every year, an estimated 15 million babies are born preterm (before 37 weeks), and this number is rising.
2. Preterm birth complications are the leading cause of death among children under 5 years old and were responsible for approximately 1 million deaths in 2015.[137]
3. Three-quarters of these deaths could be prevented with current, cost-effective interventions.
4. Across 184 countries, the rate of preterm birth ranges from 5–18% of babies born. Many preterm delivery survivors face a lifetime of disability, including learning disabilities and visual and hearing problems.

Unfortunately, both famine and feast may also affect the number of nephrons you develop before birth. Nephron numbers appear to be susceptible to even minor lifestyle choices such as Ramadan-type fasting. If the month of Ramadan occurs at the most vulnerable time in the early third trimester, this may lead to reduced and delayed kidney development and reduced nephron number.[138] When resources in the womb are restricted, they will go to development of the brain and heart.[139] After birth, there can be a far more lasting effect on longevity and risk of developing chronic kidney disease.

A study in Israel of 1,521,501 people showed that any kidney disease during childhood—even mild diseases, such as post-infectious glomerulonephritis (infection of a completely different area like the skin and throat, which causes the filters in the kidneys to swell)—and congenital anomalies of the kidneys and urinary tract, such as vesico-ureteric reflux (in which urine flows backward from the bladder into the kidneys), resulted in a fourfold increase of kidney failure under the age of 40.[140] This legacy of childhood kidney disease otherwise deemed to be relatively benign is indeed disturbing.[141] In more recent years, the risk of kidney failure was far greater in the Israeli study if the kidney disease occurred during childhood.[142] Reducing the intake of sodium is a major priority for Israel's government.[143]

Note: There are some rare kidney disorders with salt wasting for which this recommendation of salt restriction does not apply.

## Kidney health, heart health and salt

High salt intake may lead to a direct tissue effect on the kidneys, including glomerular overgrowth and scarring (glomeruli work as strainers at the end of the nephrons), independent of its effect on blood pressure.[144] These findings seem to be firm. What is somewhat less firm is whether restricting salt slows the progression of chronic kidney disease—especially in childhood, where the most common cause of end-stage kidney disease is kidney birth defects (where salt is wasted due to the small number of nephrons). Two meta-analysis studies relay a clear message: Moderate salt restriction significantly reduces blood pressure and albumin in the urine in patients with chronic kidney disease who are not yet on dialysis.[145] Salt restriction may also reduce the cardiovascular risk.[146] It would appear that restricting salt intake is important for patients with chronic kidney diseases of various causes or those who are at risk of kidney damage, such as hypertensive or diabetic patients or even prematurely born children with low numbers of nephrons.

Kidney disease affects the heart, and vice versa. Patients with advanced chronic kidney disease often experience heart failure. Heart failure is a condition caused by a poor functioning cardiac muscle and results in poor blood flow to meet the body's needs. This results in fluid overload, leg swelling, breathlessness and fatigue. The kidneys and heart work together in a bidirectional and complex relationship: The heart pumps the blood filled with oxygen throughout the body. The kidneys clean the blood, removing waste and extra water. There's also a strong connection between kidney (renal) and cardiovascular diseases. Cardiorenal syndrome type 4 is a cardiovascular disease characterized by chronic kidney disease that leads to impaired heart function.

In a group led by my friend and collaborator Professor Christopher McIntyre, we are using magnetic resonance imaging to study the sodium content in the leg. We've found that from childhood to adulthood, the sodium content in the skin, muscle, bone and other tissues is increasing with age, and even more so in patients with impaired kidney function. This extra salt build-up can cause inflammation and may explain the bothersome symptoms often experienced by patients with advanced chronic kidney disease, such as itchiness, lethargy and restless legs.

Professor McIntyre, together with our biophysics friends at the Robarts Research Institute in London, Ontario, developed a technique to measure sodium in tissue. We found that over our lifetime, we store more sodium in our tissue. However, patients with chronic kidney disease store far more sodium in their tissue than healthy people. The difference between healthy controls and patients with advanced chronic kidney disease appears to be the highest in children. In figure 22, the sodium content in the leg shows massively increased sodium concentrations in the tissues of children with advanced chronic kidney disease compared to healthy children.

Healthy            Chronic Kidney Disease
(PedCKD01)

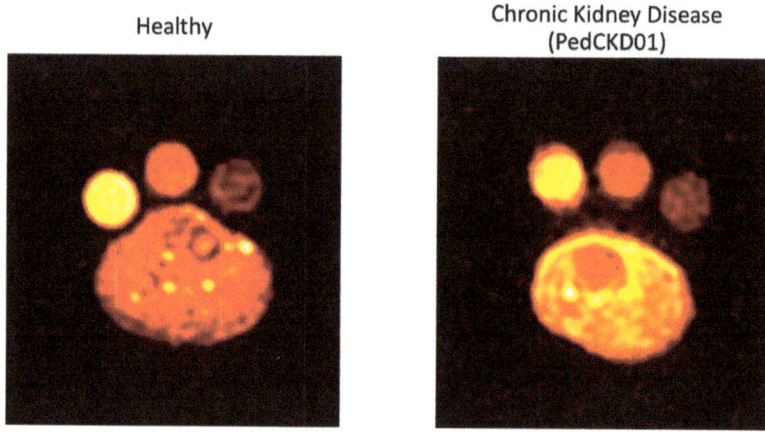

**Figure 22:** *Tissue sodium measured in a cross-section of the leg using sodium MRI technique. The figure on the left is of a healthy control; the figure on the right is from a young child with only 20% kidney function.*

If confirmed, our findings may link the connection between heart and kidney disease, and may explain why novel heart failure medications that target sodium excretion work.[147] A heart failure trial was stopped early because of the overwhelmingly beneficial effect on patient mortality when compared to the standard of care with a medication called enalapril.[148] All of this points to a pivotal role of sodium overload in both chronic kidney disease and heart failure; it should remind us about the benefit of restricting our salt consumption to below 2,300 mg per day.[149]

## Summary

The impact of lowering salt intake on chronic kidney disease is profound and appears to be independent of other factors, such as blood pressure, obesity and diabetes. The data on the reduction of end-stage kidney disease in diabetic nephropathy patients alone should convince us to forcefully introduce effective legislation that limits the salt in processed foods.[150]

# Chapter 7:
# Dementia and Salt

We learned about the impact of a high-salt diet on blood pressure. We also discussed how a high-salt diet can cause kidney stones, osteoporosis and chronic kidney disease. However, there are many other organs that may be affected as well. Much of that would be through changes related to high blood pressure, such as heart attacks and congestive heart failure. However, recent data suggests that dementia, including diseases such as Alzheimer's may be related to salt.

## What is dementia?

The term dementia is the overarching category of a set of neuropsychiatric symptoms caused by a broad variety of disorders affecting the brain. Symptoms may include difficulties with thinking, remembering, problem-solving or language that are severe enough to reduce a person's ability to perform everyday activities. A person with dementia may also experience changes in mood or behaviour. Dementia (also known as senility) is progressive, which means the symptoms will gradually get worse as more brain cells become damaged and eventually die. Dementia is not a specific disease.

Many diseases can cause dementia, including Alzheimer's disease, vascular dementia associated with strokes, and other conditions such as a head trauma with concussions, Lewy body disease, frontotemporal diseases, Creutzfeldt–Jakob disease, Parkinson's disease, Huntington's disease and others.

- **Lewy body disease**, also known as dementia associated with Lewy bodies, is a progressive dementia associated with abnormal deposits of a protein called alpha-synuclein in the brain, which affects thinking, movement, behaviour and mood.[151]

- **Frontotemporal disease** involves frontotemporal degeneration and shrinkage (atrophy). Frontotemporal disease tends to occur at a younger age than Alzheimer's disease, typically at age 40 to 45.[152] These areas of the brain are associated with personality, behaviour and language, and these conditions can have similar and overlapping symptoms.[153] The most common type is Alzheimer's disease (54%), followed by vascular dementia (16%) and others.[154]

- **Creutzfeldt–Jakob disease** is a degenerative brain disorder that progresses much more rapidly than Alzheimer's disease. It was described in association with the mad cow disease outbreak in the United Kingdom in the 1990s after eating meat from diseased cattle. However, there is a classic form that has not been linked to the sheep pellets causing mad cow disease. Creutzfeldt–Jakob disease and its variants belong to a broad group of human and animal diseases known as transmissible spongiform encephalopathies, which is characterized by spongy holes that can be seen under a microscope in affected brain tissue.[155]

- **Parkinson's disease** affects the basal ganglia of the brain and is caused by premature death of the brain cells that produce the chemical dopamine, which controls movement. Tremors, slowness and stiffness, impaired balance and muscle rigidity are the most common symptoms, but many other symptoms may be associated, including fatigue, soft speech, handwriting problems, stooped posture, constipation and debilitating sleep disturbances. While there is no cure, affected people can live with this disease for years and symptoms can be treated with medication.[156]

- **Huntington's disease** is inherited, and patients may develop symptoms typically in their thirties and forties. It has a broad impact on the functioning of a person and may include movement (involuntary jerking or writing, rigid muscles or contractures, slow or abnormal eye movement, problems with speech and swallowing), thinking (learning, lack of awareness of own behaviour, outbursts, acting without thinking, sexual promiscuity, difficulties focusing on tasks) and psychiatric disorders (insomnia, social withdrawal, irritability, fatigue and frequent thoughts about death).[157]

## How frequent is dementia?

Dementia is a major public health issue. In 2015, it was estimated that dementia affected about 50 million people around the world. About 10% of the population develops the disorder at some point in their life, and its prevalence increases with age—about 3% of people between ages 65 and 74, 19% between ages 75 and 84, and almost 50% of those over age 85.[158] And the incidence is increasing.

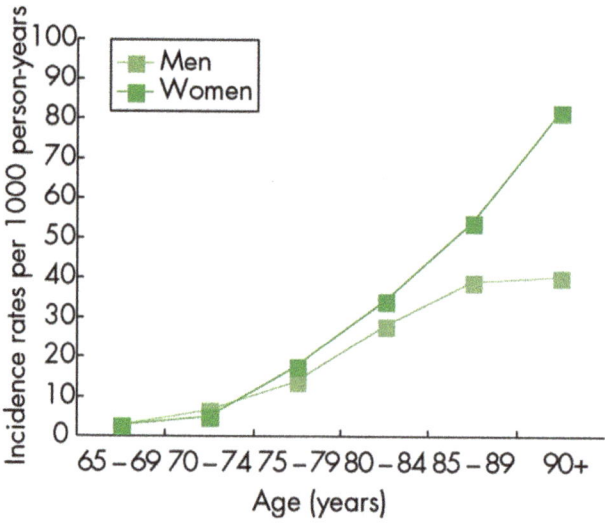

**Figure 23:** *Pooled incidence rates of dementia by sex. Based on the pooled data from eight European countries studied, there was found to be an alarming increase with age.*

In Canada today, there are over half a million Canadians living with dementia, with about 25,000 new cases diagnosed every year. By 2031, that number is expected to rise to 937,000—an increase of 66%. Canada's health care system is not equipped to deal with the staggering costs.[159] According to the Alzheimer Society of Canada, the cost is stunning: "As of 2016, the combined health-care system and out-of-pocket caregiver costs are estimated at $10.4 billion per year. By 2031, this figure is expected to increase by 60% to $16.6 billion." According to Statistics Canada, the population will grow to between 40.1 and 47.7 million by 2036.[160]

In Finland, there is a substantial problem with the number of deaths among patients with dementia. Fortunately, there has been some good progress. There is a 0.6% reduction of deaths due to dementia, although this is smaller than the 2.8% reduction in the overall mortality rate. Unfortunately, dementia still remains a major cause of death among old people in Finland (fig. 24).

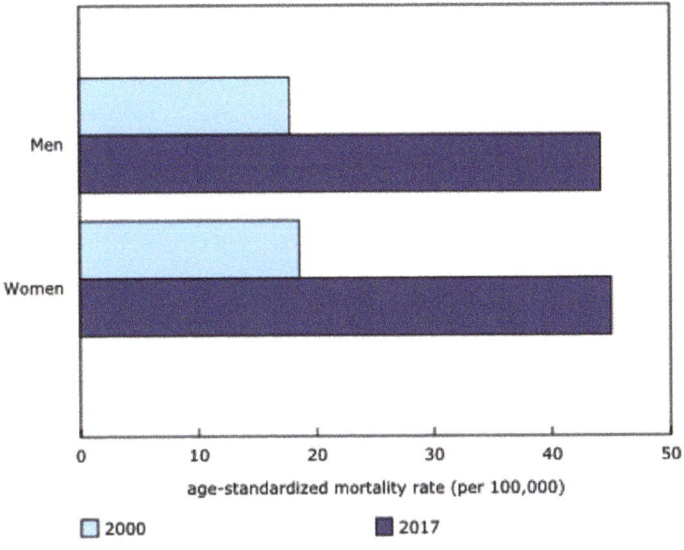

**Figure 24:** *Causes of death in Finland by age groups in 2017.*

By contrast, the mortality rates for dementia are going up tremendously in Canada. Figure 25 shows the mortality rates for dementia comparing 2000 and 2017 in Canada.

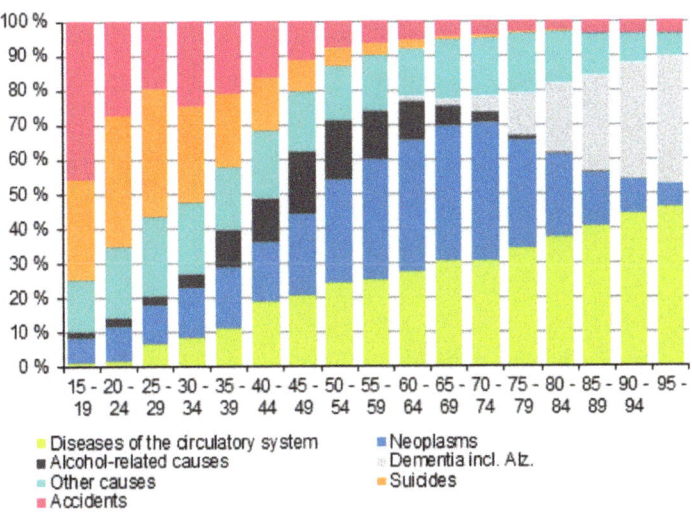

**Figure 25:** *Age-standardized mortality rate from dementia in Canada.*

It seems that the trend is vastly different between Canada and Finland, and there may indeed be a link to salt consumption. Of course, it should be highlighted that changes in the brain reflect large periods of time, and for the substantial salt consumption reduction in Finland to take effect, more time may need to pass.

## How does salt contribute to dementia?

We've already discussed dementia and high blood pressure. Remarkably, reducing salt intake by 40% in Finland resulted in an 80% drop in strokes. However, new studies have found that a high-salt diet can lead to inflammation and has been linked to dementia. Dietary salt promotes neurovascular (nerve and blood vessel) and cognitive dysfunction through an immune cell response that starts in the small intestine.[161] A number of studies found the following:

- Mice fed an equivalent of more than one teaspoon of salt per day for humans reacted by creating cells that promoted inflammation and resulted in allergic response and tissue scarring.
- Another study showed in mice and humans that sodium chloride also aggravated arthritis.[162]

While the proven blood pressure effect of how a high-salt diet can have a profound effect on the development of Alzheimer's disease is in a mouse model,[163, 164] overall, there is evidence that diet can have a profound effect on the development of Alzheimer's disease.[165] One study describes a significantly lower prevalence of dementia among Indigenous people of the Brazilian Amazon.[166] This is the area of the world with the lowest salt intake (as low as 95 mg per day). Of course, the low-salt intake is also associated with much lower cardiovascular complication rates. This data is interesting in view of a generally much higher prevalence of dementia among Indigenous populations from Canada, the United States and Australia when compared to the general population.[167] It should be pointed out that there is limited research about the epidemiology of dementia in special populations and its quality needs to be improved.

## Summary

Dementia is a major public health problem associated with an extremely high cost and use of resources. Many of the patients are in hospitals, which is really not an ideal place for them. The number of new cases is rising worldwide, and there are few strategies to reduce its occurrence. Our understanding of how dementia develops remains poor, and research needs to be intensified. However, reducing salt intake as a preventive measure seems to be an easy intervention. While the incidence is increasing everywhere else, the (very modest) decline of dementia in Finland is encouraging.

# Chapter 8: Vision and Salt

Poor eye health may also be linked to high salt intake. Sodium may affect two parts of the eye: the back of the eye (known as the retina) and the lens, where it can cause clouding of the lens or cataracts.

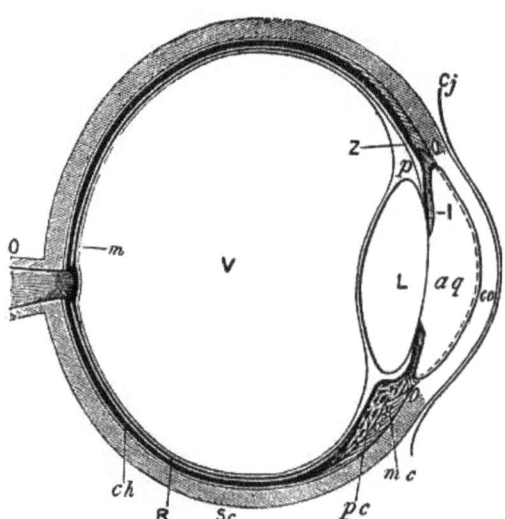

**Figure 26:** *Cross-section of an eyeball. The lens is marked as L and the retina (also known as the macula) is marked as R.*

Visual impairment is a true public health issue. About 5.7% of Canadian adults have visual impairment.[168] There are multiple factors, including smoking, high blood pressure, diabetes and memory problems. Some of the most prevalent causes are cataracts (most common), glaucoma (a condition of increased pressure within the eyeball) and macular degeneration (a degenerative condition affecting the central part of the retina—the macula—resulting in distortion or loss of central vision). At least two of the most prevalent conditions may substantially benefit from a reduction of dietary salt intake: cataracts and macular degeneration.

## Cataracts

A cataract is the clouding of the lens in the eye, which for obvious reasons leads to a decrease in vision. Cataracts often develop slowly and can affect one or both eyes. Symptoms may include faded colours, blurry or double vision, halos around light, trouble with bright lights and trouble seeing at night.[169] Reading, driving and face recognition may also be a problem. Cataracts cause about 50% of all cases of blindness and 33% of impaired vision worldwide.[170]

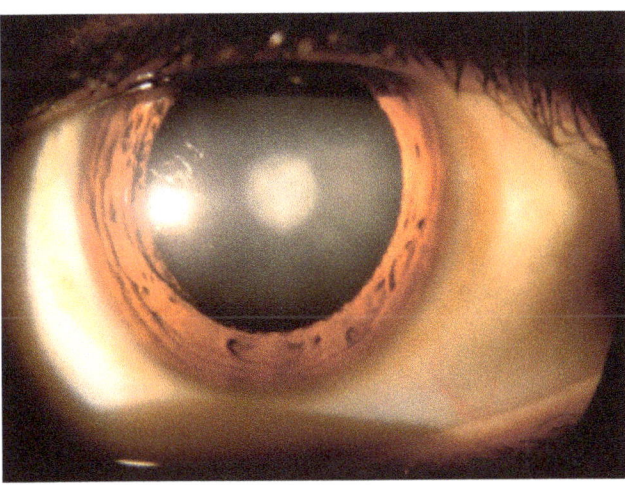

**Figure 27:** *A typical cataract. Magnified view of a cataract as seen on an examination with a slit lamp in the office of an ophthalmologist; you can see the milky discolouration of the lens.*

WHO states that cataracts are responsible for 51% of world blindness as of 2010.[171] In 2019 in the United States, 24.5 million people were affected by cataracts, which is about 7.4% of the population.[172] That same year in Canada, 3.5 million people had cataracts, or 9.4% of the population.

Of course, the causes of cataracts are multiple and complex. Former or current smoking, asthma or chronic bronchitis and cardiovascular disease all significantly increase the risk of cataracts. Studies have shown some drugs, such as chlorpromazine and corticosteroids, may cause cataracts.[173] Taking a vitamin supplement may be an important strategy to lower the incidence of cataracts. In a study of 3,089 participants, the five-year risk for cataracts was 60% lower for those who reported taking multivitamins or any supplement containing vitamin C or E for more than 10 years.[174] Other risks for developing cataracts include ultraviolet light, diabetes, high blood pressure and genetics.[175, 176]

## Cataracts and salt

Importantly, salt intake has also been linked to cataract formation. In a large study of over 22,000 Korean adults, having low income, low educational achievement and high sodium intake were significantly associated with cataract formation.[177] In a smaller study from Australia, a similar trend was observed.[178] Other studies have not conclusively demonstrated the origin of cataracts due to high sodium intake, but they do show a marked imbalance of sodium to potassium in the aqueous part of the eye and in the lens that was significantly associated with formation of cataracts.[179, 180] It may well be that other factors play an additional role. In a recent Iranian study of 97 cataract patients and a control group twice as large, it was found that higher meat intake was associated with cataract formation.[181]

## The cost of cataracts

The economic impact of cataracts is substantial. Fortunately, surgical procedures are helpful, and cataracts can be removed. In Canada, the most frequently performed surgery is cataract removal. The surgery consists of surgically removing the lens and implanting an artificial one. In 2017, the average cost of refractive lens exchange in the United States was $3,599 USD.[182] While health care insurance covers the procedure in Canada, there are lengthy wait lists. Special feature implants, specialized diagnostics and certain lasers are not insured and add additional costs.[183] In Australia, vision disorders amounted to $9.8 billion AU, while direct health care costs were $1.8 billion.[184] Even a developed nation like Australia cannot afford avoidable vision loss.

## Macular degeneration

The macula is the part of the retina responsible for central vision. Macular degeneration is a medical condition that may result in blurred or no vision in the centre of the visual field (where the best vision normally is). Often, there are no early symptoms of macular degeneration, just gradually worsening vision that may affect one or both eyes. While it does not result in complete blindness, loss of central vision can make it difficult to recognize faces, drive, read or perform other activities of daily life.[185] It typically occurs in older age. There are two different forms of age-related macular degeneration. Dry macular degeneration causes changes of the pigmented layer of the retina (retinal pigment epithelium), typically visible as dark pinpoint areas. It can start in one eye and then affect the other. You may have difficulty with central vision or seeing colours and fine details. This can progress to wet macular degeneration. Wet macular degeneration causes blurred vision and a blind spot in your vision. It occurs when abnormal blood vessels grow into the retina, making the retina "wet" (a process called choroidal neovascularization).

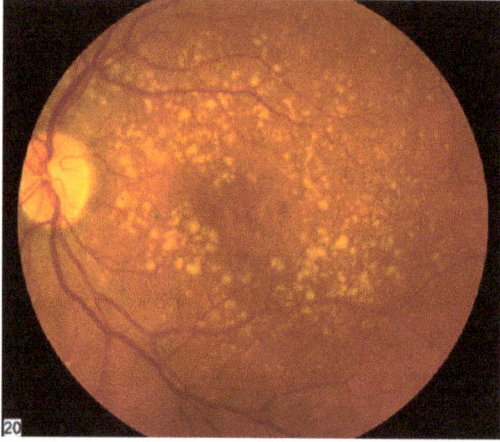

**Figure 28:** *Typical background of the eye with macular degeneration. The fundus (back portion of the eye that includes the retina and macula) showing intermediate age-related macular degeneration.*

Like cataracts, this disorder has multiple factors responsible for its development. Genetic factors may play a role.[186] Exercising, eating well and not smoking help prevent this condition. In contrast to cataract formation, antioxidant vitamins do not appear to be helpful.[187] The linkage to salt intake is largely defined through high blood pressure. Systemic high blood pressure is a risk factor of age-related retinal diseases such as diabetic retinopathy and age-related macular degeneration.

In an article about the intake of dietary salt and drinking water, and the implications for age-related macular degeneration, Andreas Bringmann and colleagues conclude: "Systemic hypertension is a risk factor of age-related retinal diseases such as diabetic retinopathy and age-related macular degeneration. High intake of dietary salt and low intake of water increase extracellular osmolality resulting in hypertension, in particular in salt-sensitive individuals."[188] Keeping oneself well hydrated is not only common sense but appears to be a very beneficial part of healthy living to prevent macular degeneration.

## Summary

There are clear associations between high salt intake and the risk of cataract formation, high blood pressure and macular degeneration. It seems prudent to reduce our salt intake and consider a healthy diet rich in vitamin C and E (or taking vitamin supplements) to reduce the financial and social impact of this major public health problem.

# Chapter 9:
# Cardiovascular Health and Salt

We've seen many benefits that should encourage you to eat a low-sodium diet—the 80% reduction of strokes in Finland is profound. There is also a benefit regarding brain aneurysms, weakened blood vessel walls that develop a bulge. The processes are the same as for vascular dementia and strokes. When the bulge in the arteries ruptures, there is a life-threatening brain bleed.[189] There is also a benefit for memory, as high blood pressure (a potential result of a high-salt diet) can affect the blood flow to the memory centres of the brain. Switching to a low-sodium diet will reduce bloating and swelling. Reducing the sodium intake to less than 1,500 mg per day is the perfect recipe for a longer life.

Let's look at salt's effect on cholesterol, heart attack and congestive heart failure.

## Cholesterol and salt

Studies are clear that a lower-salt diet significantly reduces blood pressure in people of all races, but does it lower cholesterol? Those opposed to the world-wide salt reduction campaign usually cite a meta-analysis by Niels Graudal and colleagues. In their analysis, it was found that, as a side effect of lower salt intake, certain hormones such as renin, aldosterone, noradrenaline and adrenaline increased significantly. These stress hormones may increase fatty substances in the blood, such as cholesterol and triglycerides.

However, the increase of cholesterol is largely due to an increase of low-density lipoprotein cholesterol (LDL), a transport protein responsible for transporting fat molecules in blood and tissue fluid to cells.[190] LDL is not bad cholesterol; it is an essential transport system for lipids that the human body needs to survive. There are both large and small particle LDLs, and while only the small particle is associated with cholesterol-related issues, neither is bad. Even small LDLs are necessary to transport nutrients to vessels that large LDLs cannot reach. Some fractions of LDL cholesterol, namely small dense LDL and glycated LDL, are associated with atherosclerosis (plaque build-up in the arteries) if it is oxidized within the walls of the arteries.[191]

At first glance, this modest increase of LDL cholesterol with reduced salt diet may be disturbing. However, the increase in cholesterol in the low-salt group seemed mainly due to an increase in low-density lipoprotein, which was only borderline significant. The slight decrease in high-density lipoprotein in the low-salt group was not significant—small dense and glycated LDL were not even measured. Most patients don't even get their LDL measured. In a lipid profile that your health provider may order, typically only total cholesterol, triglycerides and high-density lipoprotein cholesterol are measured.[192]

In another study, which specifically focused on this matter, and which involved the Dietary Approaches to Stop Hypertension (DASH) diet, there was no effect on blood lipid concentrations or cholesterol. The DASH diet increases intake of fruits, vegetables and low-fat dairy products, and reduces intake of saturated and total fat.[193]

Neither study accounted for obesity, which significantly affects cholesterol levels. In a recent study of 3,294 adults, after controlling for obesity, it was found there was no significant association between salt intake and lipid profiles (which include cholesterol levels).[194] The authors of the study stated:

> The study clearly demonstrated that the association between salt intake and risk factors related to cardiovascular disease is highly affected by adjustment for obesity measures,

irrespective of how obesity is measured. The associations with blood pressure were markedly attenuated when adjusting for measures of obesity and the associations with blood lipids were also highly affected. Thus, this study raises an important question about how to handle obesity measures when evaluating associations between salt intake and cardiovascular outcomes. [195]

So, what's the real story about all of this? Lower salt intake leads to reduced body water content, and in an attempt to revert the plasma volume, epinephrine, renin and angiotensin increase. These hormones inhibit insulin, which promotes insulin resistance (especially in obese subjects); as a consequence, high insulin levels compromise lipid metabolism, which increases blood cholesterol. The effects only occur in people with excess weight; there is no such relationship in people with normal weight.[196] Unfortunately, no existing study has controlled for food intake, which also strongly affects cholesterol levels. At this point in time, there is no evidence for a clear effect of salt intake and cholesterol levels.

## Heart attacks and salt

While the impact of salt intake on cholesterol levels is unclear, there is strong evidence that increased salt intake increases the risk of heart attacks.[197] This is largely due to the effect of salt restriction on blood pressure. It was shown in Finland that decreasing salt consumption by one-third decreased blood pressure, stroke rates (80%) and coronary heart disease deaths (75%).[198] Salt intake may also have a direct effect on heart and kidney health, as increased sodium leads to severe structural and functional cardiovascular and kidney abnormalities in adults with high blood pressure.[199] In a retirement home study in the United States, 1,981 elderly men were given either a potassium-enriched salt diet or a diet with regular salt intake. After 31 months, the elderly men on a potassium-enriched salt diet had a 41% decrease in cardiovascular disease death. They also lived almost 4 to 11 months longer and spent $426 USD less per year on inpatient care for cardiovascular disease.[200]

Evidence is mounting that restricting salt intake and increasing potassium intake decreases cardiovascular disease and death. Modelling studies suggest that a small reduction in dietary salt would result in a health benefit to a sizable general population. However, while countries like the United Kingdom and especially Finland have been successful in reducing salt intake, there appears to be no such trend in the United States and almost the entire population exceeds the guideline recommendations (eating less than 2,300 mg of sodium or a little more than one teaspoon of salt per day).[201]

## Congestive heart failure and salt

Another benefit of reduced salt intake is the prevention of congestive heart failure. Congestive heart failure occurs when your heart muscle doesn't pump blood as well as it should. Certain conditions, such as narrowed arteries in your heart (coronary heart disease) or high blood pressure, gradually leave your heart too weak or stiff to fill and pump efficiently. Symptoms include shortness of breath, sometimes even when lying down, swelling of the ankles and lower legs (edema), rapid or irregular heartbeat, exercise intolerance, fluid retention, lack of appetite and nausea.[202] It's proven that restricting sodium will improve the symptoms and can prevent this devastating disease that offers poor quality of life in advanced stages.

Risk factors for developing heart failure include: [203]

- High blood pressure
- Diabetes
- Coronary heart disease
- Sleep apnoea
- Congenital heart defects
- Valvular heart disease (damage to the heart valve)
- Viruses
- Alcohol use
- Tobacco use

- Kidney failure (through a complicated cross-talk of the kidneys and the heart called cardiorenal syndrome type IV)
- Obesity
- Non-steroidal anti-inflammatory drugs (such as ibuprofen, especially when taking concomitant diuretics)

It should be pointed out that certain diabetes drugs such as rosiglitazone and pioglitazone may be associated with an increased risk of heart failure. Health Canada issued a warning in 2002.[204] There are now changes in each drug's product monographs (the factual, scientific documentation on the drug), indicating that they should not be prescribed to patients with acute heart failure and that they should be discontinued if heart failure develops.[205]

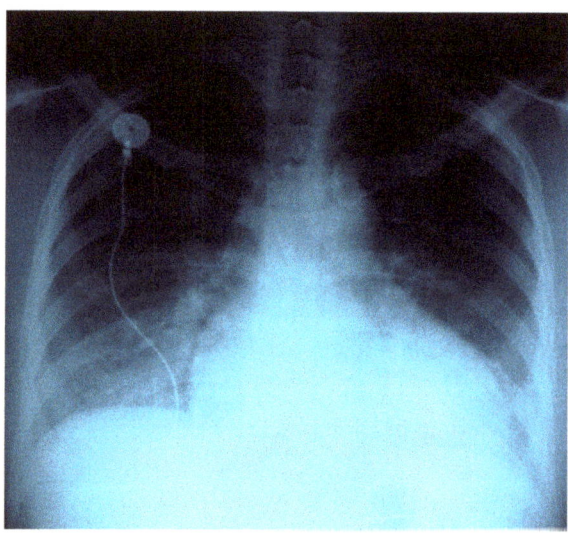

**Figure 29:** *A typical chest X-ray. This 28-year-old woman presented with congestive heart failure secondary to her chronic high blood pressure. The enlarged cardiac silhouette shows congestive heart failure due to the effects of chronic high blood pressure on the left ventricle. The heart then becomes enlarged, and fluid accumulates in the lungs (known as pulmonary congestion).*

## Summary

Salt restriction is beneficial for lowering blood pressure, reducing obesity and lowering the risk of chronic kidney disease. The many health benefits of reduced salt intake also include cardiovascular health. It is very clear that reducing salt intake is a major strategy to reduce the risk of developing congestive heart failure. Given the importance of cardiovascular health and the declining life expectancy in North America, it behoves us to reduce salt intake and incorporate better measures and policies.

# Chapter 10:
# Why was the Finnish Salt
# Campaign So Effective?

The Finnish Salt Campaign started in 1970 in Finland's far eastern province of North Karelia. The regional governor, Esa Timonen (1925–2015), appealed to the public health authorities as the government was anxious to make improvements in the health care of that province. In addition, a young physician, Dr. Pekka Puska, proposed ambitious plans, which were unproven but turned out to work well.

The situation in the North Karelia province was awful in 1970. There were a lot of early deaths and disease owing to three problems: high blood pressure, high cholesterol and excessive smoking. The problems were deeply rooted in the post Second World War situation. During the war, Finland fought against the Soviets at the Karelian border in the Winter War and the Nazis in the northernmost reaches of Lapland. Many lost their fathers. Those who returned home found a nation in transition, filled with economic problems. Veterans were awarded land by the Finnish government. Unfortunately, especially in the North Karelia province, trees were cut, and the land was used to raise cows and pigs. This caused food habits to change. Fish, game, rye bread and root vegetables were replaced by dairy and salt pork in the 1950s and 1960s. Cigarette smoking increased dramatically, a habit learned during the war. Similarly, alcohol consumption soared. All of this was in response to the scars of the war.[206] The age of smoking shifted to middle school age. As the North Karelia success story website says:

> At this crossroads of diet and drinking and depression, men began to die, young and suddenly, of cardiovascular disease. The rates in 1969—643 of 100,000 men aged 35 to 64 annually—were so striking, so high compared to the rest of the world that the public health authorities couldn't help but take note. Finland's death rates from coronary heart disease were two or even three times those of other European countries and Japan. And nowhere were they as high as where Finland had lost a frontier to the Soviet Union: the eastern province of North Karelia.[207]

The results of only two decades of these changed behaviours was a dramatic increase of community-based intervention targeting high blood pressure, high cholesterol and excessive smoking. This led to a large Finnish population study by Puska called the FINRISK Study.[208]

Interventions concentrated on a few critical points: smoking behaviour and diet, especially intake of saturated fatty acids, fibre and salt. Puska and his colleagues used a variety of tools. They set up media campaigns, community meetings, chats in people's kitchens, and carrots and sticks for farmers and food producers. They even set up village-to-village competitions for cutting back on smoking rates or reducing cholesterol levels. A crucial enabler for Puska's plan was the fact that women still ran the kitchens and controlled what made it to the dinner table. There was incredible frustration about losing husbands too soon, widowhood and bringing up fatherless children. The women took it upon themselves to lower salt, lower saturated fats and bring more vegetables to the table.

The project was highly successful. After 40 years, the cardiovascular mortality risk dropped dramatically by 75%.[209] Coronary disease mortality decreased by 82% among men and by 84% among women. These changes were profound. Two-thirds of the drop in men's mortality from stroke and half in women can be explained by the change of the three targets for intervention: smoking, salt intake and saturated fat consumption.[210] The project went national after five years, and Finland saw an 80% drop in such deaths countrywide. The changes are largely credited to Puska, a politician and member of the Finnish Parliament from 2015–2019, and the government that facilitated his work. The effort has spawned more than 1,100 related scientific publications.

However, the rest of the world did not stand still, and WHO made the reduction of salt intake a worldwide priority. Yet, we cannot copy these results in other parts of the world. We've seen the futile efforts of the Canadian government, which resulted in 84% of foods remaining over the salt limit.

In Finland, three unwavering messages were presented:

1. Reduce salt to lower blood pressure.
2. Cut saturated fats to decrease blood cholesterol numbers. Eat more produce, less meat.
3. Stop smoking.

Canada has dramatically changed its food guide.[211] Smoking rates have dropped significantly in Canada since 1999, from 25% to 13%. (But unfortunately, 2017 has seen an increase to 15%).[212] Nonetheless, cardiovascular disease and mortality rates are still increasing. Why? Because nothing has changed with regard to salt.

In Finland, the efforts eventually faded by the end of the 1980s, and it was really due to the help of legislative changes that Finland could sustain its significant reduction in salt intake. The important tools included communication, reformulation, monitoring and research. In Finland these included:

- Legislation to promote the health endeavour
- Discovery of new ways to make money from their resources, including export of their fat to consumers outside Finland
- Collaboration between the Finnish government and the food industry to replace sodium chloride with potassium citrate and other potassium salts to maintain shelf life and reduce sodium exposure

Strategies to successfully reduce population salt intake included four pillars that are proven to be effective: [213]

- Public awareness campaigns targeting consumers, food industry, decision makers, media and health professionals
- Reformulating food products, setting benchmarking targets for the food industry, adding labels and engaging the industry through motivation, cost-and-benefit analysis, consumer awareness, wide support and appealing to corporate responsibility
- Monitoring the population's salt intake by measuring urinary sodium, getting public health involved with dietary surveys, communicating reformulation progress, publishing salt content of foods, monitoring effectiveness of communication, measuring awareness of campaigns, and measuring attitudes and behaviour changes
- Research exploring a large variety of enablers and factors including epidemiology, nutrition, public health, food technology, behavioural evaluation and policy

Certainly, labels help consumers.

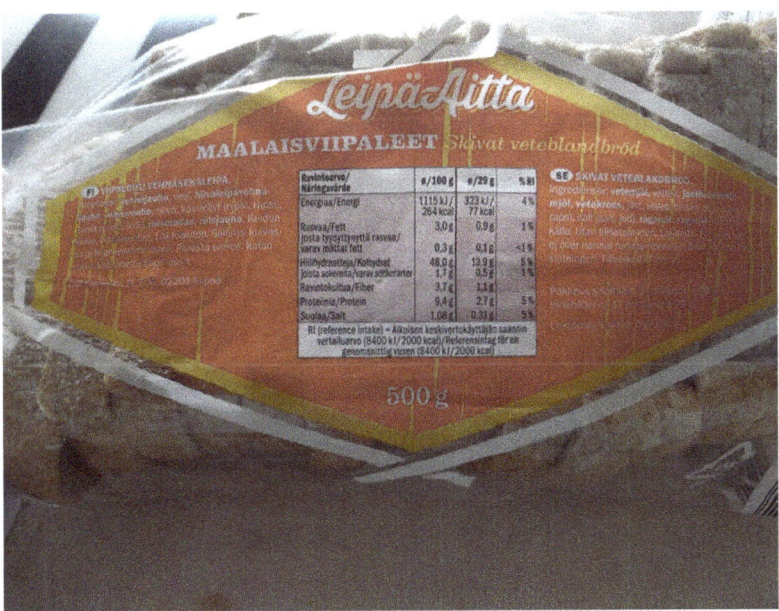

**Figure 30:** *A representative food label on a Finnish loaf of bread. A typical Finnish salt label that clearly states the percentages of the daily intake in the bottom line of the pink section.* 89

The Finnish food labels are by no means the most intelligent food labels out there. Canadian food labels introduced in 2013 look remarkably similar. British food labels combine the information with a traffic-light approach by colour coding (fig. 31). In Finland, they accomplished this by coding the colour of food with a healthy heart label and the industry competes to get that label. They also force the food industry to make unhealthy foods red for a simple signal.[214] However, the simple traffic light coding of the British food labels appears to be effective even for consumers who may be illiterate.

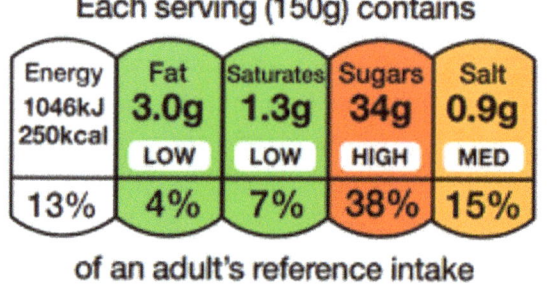

**Figure 31:** *A representative British food label.*

Labels alone, however, are not effective, as was found in Canada. I am fully aware that the process in Finland was not the result of what is listed here alone. The impact of reality shows and other public opinion makers cannot be underestimated and are difficult to measure. Nonetheless, most important are governmental tools (such as taxation in Finland), and eventually regulation and marketing control, which allows the government to fine the food industry if they exceed allowances. The latter seems to be by far the most effective tool resulting in a reduction of salt intake by 3,000 mg per day.[215]

Other countries have managed to reduce their salt intake: Lithuania by 18% (1997–2007), Japan by 17% (1977–2004), the United Kingdom by 15% (2001–2011) and Turkey by 17% (2008–2012).[216] So why are we so behind in North America? Because there are no laws in place to actually fine the food industry for exceeding healthy targets. Ultimately, we have to find champions in the legislative bodies to further the cause and push for effective legislation. Pekka Puska is now in his 70s and continues to strongly support a healthy lifestyle. It may actually be something very personal that ultimately makes people change habits.

Puska's favourite story is the following: A bus driver in Helsinki, decades after the project began, stopped his bus when he recognized Puska about to get off. "Come here!" the driver shouted. He said, "When I saw you, I decided I'll give up this," and he crushed a packet of Marlboros in his hand. Puska's passion beyond the project is obviously the people, and he seems to hold a special place for North Karelians. "North Karelians are on the lively side," he says, smiling. "We had a lot of fun."

A wide variety of tools are needed to influence reduction of salt intake, but legislative regulations on the food industry and working with the food industry to find salt alternatives appear to be the most effective tools to achieve the improvement in health seen in Finland. We need to learn from this example and adopt the Finnish salt laws. When you do not have a lot of money, this unfortunately forces you to eat processed food; those factors alone cannot and must not be the determining factor for a shorter life expectancy, a high prevalence of diabetes and poor quality of life.

As a father and a grandfather, I want my children and grandchildren to exceed my life expectancy, not to have a shorter life expectancy than my generation. It is with this in mind that I strongly advocate for stronger measures to ensure there are consequences for the food industry if they continue to add excessive salt. The voluntary approach that was chosen in Canada in 2013 is clearly not working.

# Chapter 11:
# Potential Savings

We have shown that salt is a major contributing factor for increasing disease and death associated with high blood pressure, stroke, heart attack, kidney stones, osteoporosis, dementia, cataracts, macular degeneration, heart failure and even obesity. Adopting the Finnish approach would essentially delay the onset of high blood pressure possibly by two decades and reduce strokes by 80%, heart attacks by 75% and osteoporosis-associated fractures by 50%. The impact on dementia is much more modest, but it can be argued that it may take longer than two decades to really see an improvement. The impact on cataracts is more difficult to quantify. At this point in time, there are very long wait times for cataract surgeries in Canada, especially in Ontario where numbers of those affected continue to increase.[217] Reducing the waiting time for hip replacement and cataract surgery are already provincial priorities in Ontario. What if instead of increasing capacity for cataract surgery, we reduced the development of cataracts in the first place?

It's time to consider the potential savings to our health care system. The most costly chronic disease is high blood pressure. The cost for 2019 is estimated to be $44.7 billion CAD per year. Assuming that the age of onset of high blood pressure could be pushed back from the current median age of age 40 to age 60, this would potentially cut the bill to $22.3 billion per year (see table 11-1).

In terms of acute care, cardiovascular disease was the costliest disease in Canada in 2009 ($21.2 billion in direct and indirect costs).[218] If we consider the province of Ontario as a single salt-campaign area, this could generate a potential savings of $11.1 trillion (assuming that four-sevenths of the population of Canada lives in Ontario and there is a 75% reduction of heart attacks as in Finland).[219]

Savings related to chronic kidney disease in Canada could amount to $8.9 billion per year, and for Ontario, $5.1 billion per year. Even a modest 2.6% reduction of dementia-associated mortality rate in the province would result in a cost reduction of $164.9 million, more than enough to cover the deficits of the university hospitals in Ontario.

What about strokes? The most profound improvement in Finland was an 82% reduction in strokes. According to a sensitivity analysis in 1995, the total cost of strokes in Ontario was $847 million.[220] When applying a similar approach with an annualized increase of inflation by 2.24%, this would amount to a savings of $1.1 billion per year.

What about the cost of osteoporosis-related factors? For hip fractures, there was an observed reduction of 50% in Finland. For Canada as a whole, the cost savings would amount to $88.5 million (using data for the year 2007). After adjustment for inflation, which on average is 2.24%, and adjusting for the population of Ontario, this would amount to savings of $284.9 million in the province.[221]

The estimated cost for kidney stones in the United States in 2000 was $2.1 billion USD. There are ten times more Americans than Canadians, and four-sevenths of Canadians live in Ontario. Assuming a 50% reduction of kidney stones, this would amount to annual savings of $85.5 million in Ontario. This is likely a substantial underestimate.

When you look at all the diseases together, there are potential savings of almost $40.2 billion for the province of Ontario alone. Imagine what salt reduction could save in health care costs for the whole country.

**Table 11-1:** Potential savings for high blood pressure, cardiovascular disease, chronic kidney disease, stroke, hip fractures, dementia and kidney stones in the province of Ontario

| Field | Year | Inflation adjustment | Raw cost savings ($ million) | Cost savings Ontario 2019 ($ million) |
|---|---|---|---|---|
| High blood pressure | 2019 | 1.00 | $22,350.0 | $22,350.0 |
| Cardiovascular disease | 2009 | 1.22 | 21,200.0 | 11,120.9 |
| Chronic kidney disease | 2019 | 1.00 | 8,924.0 | 5,099.4 |
| Stroke | 1995 | 1.54 | 847.0 | 1,068.0 |
| Hip fractures | 2007 | 1.27 | 224.5 | 284.9 |
| Dementia | 2016 | 1.07 | 270.4 | 164.9 |
| Kidney stones | 2000 | 1.43 | $149.7 | $85.5 |
| **Total** | | | | **$40,273.6** |

As of June 30, 2019, the Government of Ontario projected a deficit of $10.3 billion in 2019/20, unchanged from the outlook presented in the 2019 budget.[222] The Ford administration made substantial cuts to improve the budget. It's amazing that we only look at cuts in services and never consider the interconnectedness of everything. A government official told me a few years ago that the budget of the Ontario Ministry of Health for disease prevention was only $1.0 million. Admittedly, there are additional funds for public health; however, the simple change of legislated salt content in processed food and restaurant food could save almost four times more than the current budget shortfall.

A reduction of salt intake decreases blood pressure and strokes. It is effective in both genders, at any age and in any ethnic group, and effective in high-, medium- and low-income groups. The Finnish data has shown that salt reduction programs are both feasible and effective. WHO embraced salt reduction in 2013 and recommends less than 2,000 mg of sodium (one tea-spoon of salt) per day. Let us settle for 2,300 mg. Yet here in North America, we are largely ineffective. We don't have appropriate policies in place. We have no laws that govern interventions, fines and other tools to force the food industry to reduce sodium chloride in processed food to an appropriate level and replace sodium chloride with potassium salts such as potassium citrate. Regulation and marketing control in Finland were by far the most powerful tools to achieve a reduction of the salt intake by 3,000 mg per day. This book hopefully serves as a powerful appeal to consider the adoption of the Finnish salt laws.

Now you might argue: What about salt sales and revenues? It turns out that salt sales in tons for highway maintenance and water conditioning exceed food grade salt sales. Revenue from food grade salt is negligible—the biggest profit is in the field of highway maintenance.[223] The impact of a moderate salt reduction on the salt industry would be negligible. You might also argue: What if consumers dislike low-salt alternatives? I'm not arguing for an immediate reduction of salt in food by 50%; it should be implemented in steps.

Research from Australia suggests that a 25% reduction in the salt content of bread can be made without the consumer noticing it. The study compared six consecutive weeks of bread with usual sodium content to six consecutive weeks of bread with 5% reductions in sodium content each week.[224] The study showed there were no differences in scores of flavours or liking the bread. If performed more slowly, consumers would not notice anything. However, we cannot count on a voluntary approach through appeals to the food industry. We need a regulatory intervention similar to what Finland has done.

Dr. Kirsten Bibbins-Domingo and colleagues made a strong appeal to do this in the United States back in 2010. In their model, just the cardiovascular benefits alone would save $24 billion USD in health care costs. The article created substantial discussion among the medical community, but not among politicians.[225, 226] Ten years have passed and, if anything, salt consumption has gone up while life expectancy continues to decline in North America. Isn't it time to consider stronger action?

# Chapter 12:
# Summary and Conclusions

While both Canada and the United States joined the 2013 worldwide World Health Organization call to action to reduce salt intake below 2,000 mg of sodium per day, we are lagging behind, and there is no evidence of an actual reduction of salt intake—despite the proven health benefits. The impact of reducing of our daily salt intake on high blood pressure, cardiovascular disease and stroke is profound. The impact on kidney stones, osteoporosis, obesity, chronic kidney disease, dementia and vision is much less known, but the evidence is equally strong. At the same time, health care costs are spiralling. The pharmaceutical industry has discovered rare diseases as an opportunity for high-cost drugs. Less than 1% of Canadians account for 42% of patented medicine sales and the costs are rising at a staggering rate.[227] This is just one element of the rising health care costs.

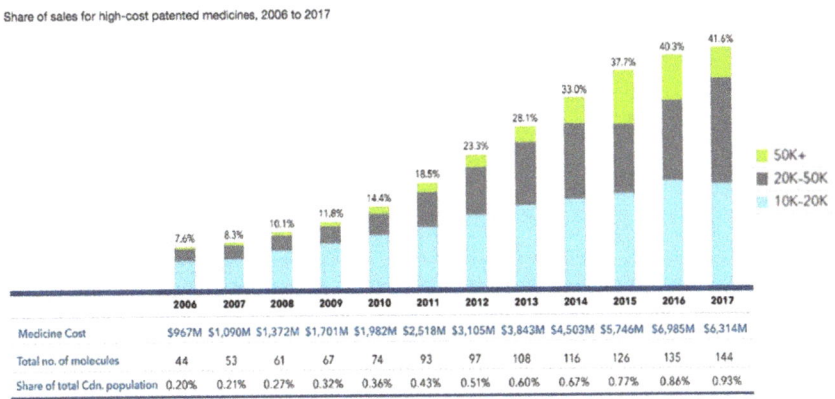

Share of sales for high-cost patented medicines, 2006 to 2017

| | 2006 | 2007 | 2008 | 2009 | 2010 | 2011 | 2012 | 2013 | 2014 | 2015 | 2016 | 2017 |
|---|---|---|---|---|---|---|---|---|---|---|---|---|
| Medicine Cost | $967M | $1,090M | $1,372M | $1,701M | $1,982M | $2,518M | $3,105M | $3,843M | $4,503M | $5,746M | $6,985M | $6,314M |
| Total no. of molecules | 44 | 53 | 61 | 67 | 74 | 93 | 97 | 108 | 116 | 126 | 135 | 144 |
| Share of total Cdn. population | 0.20% | 0.21% | 0.27% | 0.32% | 0.36% | 0.43% | 0.51% | 0.60% | 0.67% | 0.77% | 0.86% | 0.93% |

**Figure 32:** *This bar graph depicts the high-cost medicine share of total patented medicine sales per year from 2006 to 2017. The bars are subdivided into three bands based on average annual costs: $10,000–20,000; $20,000–50,000; and greater than $50,000. The table below the graph gives additional information including the cost of medicine, total number of molecules and estimated treatment population as a share of the total Canadian population for each year.*

The health of the population is deteriorating. Cardiovascular disease, osteoporosis, dementia, high blood pressure, chronic kidney disease, vision diseases and many more are on the rise. In this book, we've seen not only the overwhelming evidence for a benefit of a salt reduction by about 40% but also the enormous financial benefits for the health care system. Current legislative bodies are all too often focused on cuts rather than prevention.

Benjamin Franklin said in fire-threatened Philadelphia back in 1736: "An ounce of prevention is worth a pound of cure."[228] So many diseases are interconnected. A single change can have profound benefits. We have seen in Finland how 40% salt reduction can work. The legislative and regulatory approach of the Finnish government made it successful. The Canadian government's 2013 appeal to the food industry proved ineffective. It is time for politicians to consider much harder actions and regulatory initiatives to crack down on the reckless over-salting of our processed food. This can be done in steps that are not noticeable to the public. Alternatives such as potassium citrate will achieve a similar shelf life while having additional health benefits.

I strongly urge the governments of this world to adopt the Finnish salt laws to improve the health and the longevity of their citizens. The WHO appeal to cut salt intake must be implemented with some force; the food industry will rarely do this voluntarily. The reduction of salt through legislation and intervention is feasible, effective, safe and without significant economic consequences.

As a father and grandfather, it is unacceptable to me that the life expectancy of our young generation may be as much as five years shorter than that of the boomer generation.[229] Let us look to the future for better health and longevity. We need to reduce our consumption of salt. It is time for action!

# Acknowledgments

First and foremost, I would like to thank Dr. Maria E. Diaz-Gonzalez de Ferris, MD, MPH, PhD, for the very careful edits of the entire book. She is Professor and Director of the Healthcare Transition program at the University of North Carolina at Chapel Hill. Not only did Maria carefully review everything, she also changed the readability level and went over every part of the manuscript. She also is the dear friend and personal motivator who kept me on target. I further express my gratitude to Ms. Savanah Rae Duncan, MBA student in London, Ontario, and personal assistant, for the critical and detailed review and editing of all aspects of the book. She also collated all the literature for the chapter on current salt legislation and obtained permissions for the figures. I thank Mr. Jamie Ollivier from Victoria, British Columbia, for suggesting the title. I also want to thank Dr. Carmen Inés Rodriguez Cuellar from Bogota and Dr. Golbon Foroughi from New York for their critical review.

Most importantly, I dedicate this book to my parents, Ute Annemarie Roswitha Filler and Hans Richard Karl Filler, Dipl. sc. pol., from Goslar, Germany, and to my children, Eva, Thies, Reenste and Hannes. Without their support, this book would have never been completed in a timely manner.

# Endnotes

## Introduction

1   Sara Chodosh, "The CDC knows why U.S. life expectancy keeps dropping—but no one knows how to stop it: three things are shortening American lives," *Popular Science*, last modified October 31, 2019, https://www.popsci.com/life-expectancy-declining (accessed October 6, 2019).

2   Laura Santhanam, "American life expectancy has dropped again. Here's why," *PBS News Hour*, November 9, 2018, https://www.pbs.org/newshour/health/american-life-expectancy-has-dropped-again-heres-why (accessed October 6, 2019).

3   "Healthiest countries 2020," *World Population Review*, October 25, 2019, http://worldpopulationreview.com/countries/healthiest-countries/ (accessed September 6, 2019).

## Chapter 1: Current Salt Legislation in Developed Countries

4   Francisco Apellániz, "Venetian trading networks in the medieval Mediterranean," *Journal of Interdisciplinary History* 44, no. 2 (Autumn, 2013): 157–179, https://www.mitpressjournals.org/doi/pdf/10.1162/JINH_a_00535.

5   "Salt reduction: key facts," *World Health Organization*, June 30, 2016, https://www.who.int/news-room/fact-sheets/detail/salt-reduction (accessed September 16, 2019).

6   "Salt reduction: key facts," WHO.

7   "Salt reduction: key facts." WHO.

8   "A comprehensive global monitoring framework including indicators and a set of voluntary global targets for the prevention and control of noncommunicable diseases," second WHO discussion paper, World Health Organization (March 22, 2012), accessed June 27, 2014, http://www.who.int/nmh/events/2012/discussion_paper2_20120322.pdf.

9   Lorena Allemandi et al., "Sodium content in processed foods in Argentina: compliance with the national law," *Cardiovascular Diagnosis and Therapy* 5, no. 3 (June 2015), https://www.ncbi.nlm.nih.gov/pmc/articles/PMC4451319/ (accessed September 16, 2019).

10   Sarah Roache, "World salt awareness week: innovative regulations to reduce salt intake," Georgetown University, *O'Neill Institute for National and Global Health Law* (February 27, 2017), https://oneill.law.georgetown.edu/worldsaltawarenessweek/ (accessed September 16, 2019).

11   Bruce Neal, Wu Yangfeng and Nicole Li, "The effectiveness and costs of population interventions to reduce salt consumption," World Health Organization (Geneva, Switzerland, 2007), https://www.who.int/dietphysicalactivity/Neal_saltpaper_2006.pdf (accessed July 10, 2019).

12   "Salt reduction: Key facts," WHO.

13   Alexander A. Leung et al., "Hypertension Canada's 2016 Canadian hypertension education program guidelines for blood pressure measurement, diagnosis, assessment of risk, prevention, and treatment of hypertension," *Canadian Journal of Cardiology* 32, no. 5 (May 1, 2016): 569–88.

14   JoAnne Arcand et al., "Results of a national survey examining Canadians' concern, actions, barriers, and support for dietary sodium reduction interventions," *Canadian Journal of Cardiology* 29, no. 5 (May 1, 2013): 628–31.

15   "Sodium reduction in processed foods in Canada: an evaluation of progress toward voluntary targets from 2012 to 2016," *Government of Canada*, https://www.canada.ca/en/health-canada/services/food-nutrition/legislation-guidelines/guidance-documents/guidance-food-industry-reducing-sodium-processed-foods-progress-report-2017.html (accessed July 10, 2019).

16   Lawrence J. Appel, "Salt reduction in the United States: halve salt in processed and restaurant food, says American Medical Association," *BMJ* 333, no. 7568 (September 16, 2006): 561–2, https://www.ncbi.nlm.nih.gov/pmc/articles/PMC1569959/ (accessed September 16, 2019).

17   "Benefits of US salt reduction strategy to US food industry," University of Liverpool, *ScienceDaily*,   https://www.sciencedaily.com/releases/2019/07/190724103944.htm (accessed September 16, 2019).

## Chapter 2: Kidney Stones and Salt

18   The typical teen consumes 3,310 (±70 standard error of the mean) milligrams (mg) of sodium per day. "What we eat in America, DHHS-USDA dietary survey integration," United States 2007–2008 data, National Health and Nutrition Examination Survey, *Centers for Disease Control and Prevention*, https://www.cdc.gov/nchs/nhanes/wweia.htm (accessed September 16, 2019).

19   "Sodium in Canada," *Government of Canada*, https://www.canada.ca/en/health-canada/services/food-nutrition/healthy-eating/sodium.html (accessed June 12, 2019).

20   "Salt reduction: key facts." WHO.

21   Carmen Inés Rodriguez Cuellar et al., "Educational review: role of the pediatric nephrologists in the work-up and management of kidney stones," *Pediatric Nephrology* 35, no. 3 (January 4, 2019): 383–97, https://www.ncbi.nlm.nih.gov/pubmed/30607567.

22   "Sodium food sources in the Canadian diet," https://www.canada.ca/en/health-canada/services/food-nutrition/healthy-eating/sodium/research/sodium-food-sources-canadian-diet.html (accessed June 12, 2019).

23   "Healthiest countries 2020," *World Population Review*.

24   Tsering Dhondup et al., "Risk of ESRD and mortality in kidney and bladder stone formers," *American Journal of Kidney Diseases* 72, no. 6 (December 6, 2018): 790–7, https://www.ncbi.nlm.nih.gov/pubmed/30146423.

25   Ajay P. Sharma and Guido Filler, "Epidemiology of pediatric urolithiasis," *Indian Journal of Urology* 26, no. 4 (October 2010): 516–22, https://www.ncbi.nlm.nih.gov/pubmed/21369384.

26   Elaine M. Worcester and Fredric Coe, "Calcium kidney stones," *New England Journal of Medicine* 363 (September 2, 2010): 954–63, https://www.nejm.org/doi/full/10.1056/NEJMcp1001011.

27   Charles D. Scales Jr. et al., "Prevalence of kidney stones in the United States," *European Urology* 62, no. 1 (July 2012):160–5, https://www.ncbi.nlm.nih.gov/pubmed/22498635.

28   Kirsten Kusumi, Brian Becknell and Andrew Schwaderer, "Trends in pediatric urolithiasis: patient characteristics, associated diagnoses, and financial burden," *Pediatric Nephrology* 30, no. 5 (May 2015): 805–10, https://www.ncbi.nlm.nih.gov/pubmed/25481020.

29   "Healthiest countries 2020."

30   "Salt reduction: key facts." WHO.

31   Margaret S. Pearle, Elizabeth A. Calhoun and Gary C. Curhan, "Urologic diseases in America project: urolithiasis," American Urological Association, *Journal of Urology* 173 (2005): 848–57, https://www.auajournals.org/article/S0022-5347(05)60357-6/abstract.

32   "Salt reduction: key facts." WHO.

33   David J. Sas et al., "Increasing incidence of kidney stones in children evaluated in the emergency department," *Journal of Pediatrics* 157, no. 1 (July 2010): 132–7, https://www.jpeds.com/article/S0022-3476(10)00110-1/fulltext.

34   "Salt reduction: key facts." WHO.

35   Jodi A. Antonelli et al., "Use of the National Health and Nutrition Examination Survey to calculate the impact of obesity and diabetes on cost and prevalence of urolithiasis in 2030," *European Urology* 66, no. 4 (2014): 724–9, https://www.ncbi.nlm.nih.gov/pmc/articles/PMC4227394/.

36   Gregory E. Tasian et al., "Annual incidence of nephrolithiasis among children and adults in South Carolina from 1997 to 2012," *Clinical Journal of American Society Nephrology* 11, no. 3 (March 7, 2016): 488–96, https://www.ncbi.nlm.nih.gov/pubmed/26769765.

37   Jane E. Henney, Christine L. Taylor and Caitlin S. Boon, eds., "Strategies to reduce sodium intake in the United States," Institute of Medicine Committee (National Academies Press: Washington, April 2010).

38   Catherine M. Loria et al., "Usual sodium intakes compared with current dietary guidelines—United States, 2005–2008," Morbidity and Mortality Weekly Report, *Centers for Disease Control and Prevention* 60, no. 41 (October 21, 2011): 1413–7, https://www.cdc.gov/mmwr/preview/mmwrhtml/mm6041a1.htm.

39   Alanna Moshfegh et al., "Vital signs: food categories contributing the most to sodium consumption—United States, 2007–2008," Morbidity and Mortality Weekly Report, *Centers for Disease Control and Prevention* 61, no. 5 (February 2012): 92–8, https://www.cdc.gov/mmwr/preview/mmwrhtml/mm6105a3.htm.

40   Peter W. Fischer et al., "Sodium food sources in the Canadian diet," *Applied Physiology, Nutrition and Metabolism* 34, no. 5 (October 2009): 884–92, https://www.ncbi.nlm.nih.gov/pubmed/19935850.

41   Rafael V. Picon et al., "Prevalence of hypertension among elderly persons in urban Brazil: a systematic review with meta-analysis," *American Journal of Hypertension* 26, no. 4 (April 2013): 541–8, https://www.ncbi.nlm.nih.gov/pubmed/23467209.

42   The more sodium you ingest, the more sodium the kidneys must get rid of, as the sodium value in the blood must be maintained in a tight range between 135–145 mmol/litre. Christopher Nordin et al., "The nature and significance of the relationship between urinary sodium and urinary calcium in women," *Journal of Nutrition* 123 (1993): 1615–22, https://www.researchgate.net/publication/14838095_The_Nature_and_Significance_of_the_Relationship_between_Urinary_Sodium_and_Urinary_Calcium_in_Women.

43   Christopher Nordin et al., "Relationship between urinary sodium and urinary calcium in women."

44   Velimir Matkovic et al., "Urinary calcium, sodium, and bone mass of young females," *American Journal of Clinical Nutrition* 62, no. 2 (August 1995): 417–25, https://www.ncbi.nlm.nih.gov/pubmed/7625351.

45   Alexies V. Osorio and Uri S. Alon, "The relationship between urinary calcium, sodium, and potassium excretion and the role of potassium in treating idiopathic hypercalciuria," *Pediatrics* 100, no. 4 (October 1997): 675–81, https://www.ncbi.nlm.nih.gov/pubmed/9310524.

46   Larisa Kovacevic et al., "From hypercalciuria to hypocitraturia—a shifting trend in pediatric urolithiasis?" *Journal of Urology* 188, supplement 4 (2012): 1623–7, https://www.ncbi.nlm.nih.gov/pubmed/22910255.

47   Deborah E. Sellmeyer, Monique Schloetter and Anthony Sebastian, "Potassium citrate prevents increased urine calcium excretion and bone resorption induced by a high sodium chloride diet," *Journal of Clinical Endocrinology and Metabolism* 87, no. 5 (May 2002): 2008–12, https://academic.oup.com/jcem/article/87/5/2008/2846608.

## Chapter 3: High Blood Pressure and Salt

48   Naomi C. Hamm et al., "Trends in chronic disease incidence rates from the Canadian Chronic Disease Surveillance System," *Health Promotion and Chronic Disease Prevention in Canada* 39, no. 6–7 (June 2019): 216–24, https://www.ncbi.nlm.nih.gov/pubmed/31210047.

49  Gulam Muhammed Al Kibria et al., "Age-stratified prevalence, treatment status, and associated factors of hypertension among US adults following application of the 2017 ACC/AHA guideline," *Hypertension Research* 42, no. 10 (October 2019) 1631–43, https://www.ncbi.nlm.nih.gov/pubmed/31160699.

50  Paul K. Whelton et al., "2017 ACC/ AHA/ AAPA/ ABC/ ACPM/ AGS/ APhA/ ASH/ ASPC/ NMA/ PCNA guideline for the prevention, detection, evaluation, and management of high blood pressure in adults: a report of the American College of Cardiology/American Heart Association Task Force on clinical practice guidelines," *Hypertension* 71, no. 6 (June 2018): e13–115, https://www.ahajournals.org/doi/10.1161/HYP.0000000000000065.

51  Joseph T. Flynn et al., "Clinical practice guideline for screening and management of high blood pressure in children and adolescents," *Pediatrics* 140, no. 3 (September 2017): e20171904, https://pediatrics.aappublications.org/content/140/3/e20171904.

52  Ped(z) pediatric calculator, https://www.pedz.de/en/welcome.html.

53  Kristi Reynolds et al., "The utility of ambulatory blood pressure monitoring for diagnosing white coat hypertension in older adults," *Current Hypertension Reports* 17, no. 11 (November 2015): 86, https://www.ncbi.nlm.nih.gov/pmc/articles/PMC4687733/.

54  Joseph T. Flynn et al., "Update: ambulatory blood pressure monitoring in children and adolescents: a scientific statement from the American Heart Association," *Hypertension* 63, no. 5 (May 2014): 1116–35, https://www.ncbi.nlm.nih.gov/pubmed/24591341.

55  John F. Nunn, "Ancient Egyptian medicine," *Transactions of the Medical Society of London* 113 (1996): 57–68.

56  Nima Ghasemzadeh and A. Maziar Zafari, "A brief journey into the history of the arterial pulse," *Cardiology Research and Practice* 2011 (July 28, 2011): 164832, https://www.hindawi.com/journals/crp/2011/164832/.

57  Jeremy Booth, "A short history of blood pressure measurement," *Proceedings of the Royal Society of Medicine* 70, no. 11 (November 1977): 793–9, https://www.ncbi.nlm.nih.gov/pmc/articles/PMC1543468/.

58  Bruce Neal, Wu Yangfeng and Nicole Li, "The effectiveness and costs of population interventions."

59  H. Cook and J. Briggs, "Clinical observations of blood pressure," *Johns Hopkins Hospital Reports* 11 (1903): 451–534.

60  "Salt reduction: key facts." WHO.

61   Ariel Roguin, "Scipione Riva-Rocci and the men behind the mercury sphyg-momanometer," *International Journal of Clinical Practice* 60, no. 1 (January 2006): 73–9, https://onlinelibrary.wiley.com/doi/abs/10.1111/j.1742-1241.2005.00548.x.

62   Guido Filler and Ajay P. Sharma, "Methodology of casual blood pressure measurement," *Pediatric Hypertension* (January 2017): 1–17, https://www.researchgate.net/publication/318152267_Methodology_of_Casual_Blood_Pressure_Measurement.

63   Elizabeth B. Kirkland et al., "Trends in healthcare expenditures among US adults with hypertension: national estimates, 2003–2014," *Journal of the American Heart Association* 7, no. 11 (May 30, 2018): e008731, https://www.ncbi.nlm.nih.gov/pubmed/29848493.

64   Sundeep Mishra, "Diuretics in primary hypertension—reloaded," *Indian Heart Journal* 68, no. 5 (September–October 2016): 720–3, https://www.ncbi.nlm.nih.gov/pubmed/27773415.

65   Conventional wisdom has suggested that we cannot grow new brain cells after birth, but this is not the case. While most brain cells are formed in the womb until 36 weeks of gestation, certain parts of the brain continue to make neural (brain) cells. The prefrontal cortex, for instance, continues to mature well into your twenties. The prefrontal cortex is the cerebral cortex covering the front part of the frontal lobe (forehead). This brain region has been implicated in planning complex cognitive behaviour, personality expression, decision making and moderating social behaviour. Perhaps the most striking example is plasticity of the human brain, also known as neuroplasticity. This term describes the constant change of the brain throughout life and its ability to transfer a given function to a different location. A case that continues to strike me is that of a now eight-year-old patient of mine. She suffered severe asphyxia at birth and multiple organ injuries. Only a small sliver of her brain was seen on a computer tomography after her discharge. The neurologists gave her a grim prognosis. Today, she walks, talks, attends school and even remembers to take her anti-rejection medications.

66   With normal aging, nephron loss occurs and results in decreased kidney function; it is called age-related decrease in the glomerular filtration rate. Aleksandar Denić et al., "The substantial loss of nephrons in healthy human kidneys with aging," *Journal of the American Society Nephrology* 28, no. 1 (January 2017): 313–20, https://www.ncbi.nlm.nih.gov/pubmed/27401688.

67   In the Mayo Clinic study of 1,638 living kidney donors, researchers obtained cortical volumes of both kidneys from pre-donation computed tomography scans. At the time of kidney transplant, they obtained and analyzed the sections of a biopsy specimen of the cortex to determine the density of both non-sclerotic (non-scarred) and globally sclerotic glomeruli; the total number of glomeruli was estimated from cortical volume × glomerular density. Donors between ages 18 and 29 had a mean

990,661 non-sclerotic glomeruli and 16,614 globally sclerotic glomeruli per kidney, which progressively decreased to 520,410 non-sclerotic glomeruli per kidney and increased to 141,714 globally sclerotic glomeruli per kidney in donors between ages 70 and 75. "What we eat in America," NHNE Survey.

68    When the treatment effect (or effect size) is consistent from one study to the next, a meta-analysis can be used to identify this common effect. A 100 mmol reduction in 24-hour urinary sodium (6 g per day of salt) was associated with a fall in systolic blood pressure of 5.8 mmHg (95%CI: 2.5 to 9.2, P=0.001), even when differences in age, ethnic group and blood pressure status were accounted for. The meta-analysis also showed that a reduction of salt intake alone to approximately 40% of the current level resulted in a reduction of the systolic blood pressure by 6.7 mmHg and 3.5 mmHg for the diastolic blood pressure. Feng J. He et al., "Effect of longer term modest salt reduction on blood pressure," *Cochrane Database of Systematic Reviews* (April 30, 2013), https://doi.org/10.1002/14651858.CD004937.pub2.

69    These changes caused a significant effect on the systolic blood pressure (pooled mean difference: 4.91 mmHg) in Finland. Heikki Karppanen and Eero Mervaala, "Sodium intake and hypertension," *Progress in Cardiovascular Diseases* 49, no. 2 (September–October 2006): 59–75, https://www.sciencedirect.com/science/article/abs/pii/S0033062006000831?via%3Dihub.

70    "Finland: salt action summary," *World Action on Salt and Health*, http://www.worldactiononsalt.com/worldaction/europe/finland/ (accessed July 8, 2019).

71    Lirije Hyseni et al. "Systematic review of dietary salt reduction policies: evidence for an effectiveness hierarchy?" *PLoS One* 12, no. 5 (May 18, 2017): e0177535, https://www.ncbi.nlm.nih.gov/pubmed/28542317.

## Chapter 4: Osteoporosis and Salt

72    Von Uwe Groenewold, "Viele patienten können keinen Staubsauger mehr durch die Wohnung ziehen," *Welt Am Sonntag*, https://www.welt.de/print-wams/article136768/Viele-Patienten-koennen-keinen-Staubsauger-mehr-durch-die-Wohnung-ziehen.html (accessed July 18, 2019).

73    Cyrus Cooper, G. Campion and L. Joseph Melton 3rd, "Hip fractures in the elderly: a world-wide projection," *Osteoporosos International* 2, no. 6 (November 1992): 285–9, https://www.ncbi.nlm.nih.gov/pubmed/1421796.

74    L. Joseph Melton 3rd et al., "Perspective: how many women have osteoporosis?" *Journal of Bone and Mineral Research* 7, no. 9 (September 1992): 1005–10, https://www.ncbi.nlm.nih.gov/pubmed/1414493.

75   A. Randell et al., "Direct clinical and welfare costs of osteoporotic fractures in elderly men and women," *Osteoporosis International* 5, no. 6 (February 1995): 427–32, https://www.researchgate.net/publication/14506266_Direct_clinical_and_welfare_costs_of_osteoporotic_fractures_in_elderly_men_and_women.

76   "The overall low bone mass prevalence was 43.9%, from which we estimated that 43.4 million older adults had low bone mass. We estimated that 7.7 million non-Hispanic White, 0.5 million non-Hispanic Black, and 0.6 million Mexican American adults had osteoporosis and another 33.8, 2.9 and 2.0 million had low bone mass, respectively. When combined, osteoporosis and low bone mass at the femoral neck or lumbar spine affected an estimated 53.6 million older US adults in 2010." In that same study, the number of people in the United States over age 50 was 99,048,838. It may mean that more than half of them have osteoporosis. Nicole C. Wright et al., "The recent prevalence of osteoporosis and low bone mass in the United States based on bone mineral density at the femoral neck or lumbar spine," *Journal of Bone and Mineral Research* 29, no. 11 (November 2014): 2520–6, https://www.ncbi.nlm.nih.gov/pmc/articles/PMC4757905/.

77   Susan Ziglar and Tracy S. Hunter, "The effect of hormonal oral contraception on acquisition of peak bone mineral density of adolescents and young women," *Journal of Pharmacy Practice* 25, no. 3 (June 2012): 331–40, https://www.ncbi.nlm.nih.gov/pubmed/22572223.

78   Léon Nshimyumukiza et al., "An economic evaluation: simulation of the cost-effectiveness and cost-utility of universal prevention strategies against osteoporosis-related fractures," *Journal of Bone and Mineral Research* 28, no. 2 (February 2013): 383–94, https://www.ncbi.nlm.nih.gov/pubmed/22991210.

79   "Fast facts," *Osteoporosis Canada*, https://osteoporosis.ca/about-the-disease/fast-facts/ (accessed October 20, 2016).

80   Jean-Eric Tarride et al., "The burden of illness of osteoporosis in Canada," *Osteoporosis International* 23, no. 11 (November 2012): 2591–2600, https://www.ncbi.nlm.nih.gov/pubmed/22398854.

81   In some countries, such as Norway, which has the highest prevalence of osteoporosis in the world, hip fracture rates are declining, likely due to strategies for prevention of falls. For Canada and the overall population, the average age-adjusted annual percentage decrease in hip fracture rates was 1.2% (95% confidence interval, 1.0%–1.3%) per year from 1985 to 1996 and 2.4% (95% confidence interval, 2.1%–2.6%) per year from 1996 to 2005 (P < .001 for difference in slopes). However, the rates remain high with 9.2 per 100,000 persons for over age 55; 43.9 per 100,000 for ages 55 to 64; 135.1 per 100,000 for ages 65 to 74; 466.2 per 100,000 for ages 75 to 84; and 1484.4 per 100,000 for over age 85. William D. Leslie et al., "Trends in hip fracture rates in Canada," *Journal of the American Medical*

*Association* 302, no. 8 (August 26, 2009): 883–9, https://jamanetwork.com/journals/jama/fullarticle/184467.

82   "What people recovering from alcoholism need to know about osteoporosis," *National Institutes of Health*, https://www.bones.nih.gov/health-info/bone/osteoporosis/conditions-behaviors/alcoholism.

83   Jeanie Lerche Davis, "Drink less for strong bones," *WebMD*, https://www.webmd.com/osteoporosis/features/alcohol#1 (accessed July 10, 2019).

84   Robert F. Klein, "Alcohol-induced bone disease: impact of ethanol on osteoblast proliferation," *Alcoholism, Clinical and Experimental Research* 21, no. 3 (May 1997): 392–9, https://www.ncbi.nlm.nih.gov/pubmed/9161596.

85   Jill A. Marrone et al., "Moderate alcohol intake lowers biochemical markers of bone turnover in postmenopausal women," *Menopause* 19, no. 9 (September 2012): 974–9, https://www.ncbi.nlm.nih.gov/pmc/articles/PMC3597753/.

86   Caterina Trevisan et al., "The impact of smoking on bone metabolism, bone mineral density and vertebral fractures in postmenopausal women," *Journal of Clinical Densitometry* (July 10, 2019): S1094-6950(19)30108-8, https://www.sciencedirect.com/science/article/abs/pii/S1094695019301088.

87   Mattias Callréus, Fiona McGuigan and Kristina Akesson, "Adverse effects of smoking on peak bone mass may be attenuated by higher body mass index in young female smokers," *Calcified Tissue International* 93, no. 6 (December 2013): 517–25, https://www.ncbi.nlm.nih.gov/pubmed/24005807.

88   Robert Rudäng et al., "Smoking is associated with impaired bone mass development in young adult men: a 5-year longitudinal study," *Journal of Bone and Mineral Research* 27, no. 10 (October 2012): 2189–97, https://asbmr.onlinelibrary.wiley.com/doi/pdf/10.1002/jbmr.1674.

89   Somaye Fatahi et al., "The association of dietary and urinary sodium with bone mineral density and risk of osteoporosis: a systematic review and meta-analysis," *Journal of the American College of Nutrition* 37, no. 6 (August 2018): 522–32, https://www.ncbi.nlm.nih.gov/pubmed/29617220.

90   Karin Wigertz et al., "Racial differences in calcium retention in response to dietary salt in adolescent girls," *American Journal of Clinical Nutrition* 81, no. 4 (April 2005): 845–50, https://academic.oup.com/ajcn/article/81/4/845/4649038.

91   Michelle Braun et al., "Racial differences in skeletal calcium retention in adolescent girls with varied controlled calcium intakes," *American Journal of Clinical Nutrition* 85, no. 6 (June 1, 2007): 1657–63, https://academic.oup.com/ajcn/article/85/6/1657/4633047.

92   There are a lot of open questions, but clearly normal vitamin D status and higher calcium intake are beneficial, whereas dietary salt increases urinary calcium wasting. Exercise can enhance the impact of a low-salt and high-calcium diet. Connie M. Weaver, "The role of nutrition on optimizing peak bone mass," *Asia Pacific Journal of Clinical Nutrition* 17, no. 1 supplement (2008): 135–7, http://apjcn.nhri.org.tw/server/APJCN/17%20Suppl%201//135.pdf.

93   Pekka Kannus et al., "Continuously declining incidence of hip fracture in Finland: analysis of nationwide database in 1970–2016," *Archives of Gerontology Geriatrics* 77 (July–August 2018): 64–7, https://www.sciencedirect.com/science/article/abs/pii/S0167494318300694.

94   Axel Svedbom et al., "Osteoporosis in the European Union: a compendium of country-specific reports," *Archives of Osteoporosis* 8, no. 1–2 (December 2013): 137, https://www.researchgate.net/publication/257647904_Osteoporosis_in_the_European_Union_A_compendium_of_country-specific_reports.

## Chapter 5: Obesity and Salt

95   Thomas R. Dawber, Gilcin F. Meadors and Felix E. Moore Jr., "Epidemiological approaches to heart disease: the Framingham Study," presented at a joint session of the epidemiology, health officers, medical care and statistics sections of the American Public Health Association, at the seventy-eighth annual meeting in St. Louis, Missouri, November 3, 1950, https://ajph.aphapublications.org/doi/pdf/10.2105/AJPH.41.3.279.

96   "Framingham Heart Study," *Wikipedia*, https://en.wikipedia.org/wiki/Framingham_Heart_Study (accessed August 15, 2019).

97   William B. Kannel, "Elevated systolic blood pressure as a cardiovascular risk factor," *American Journal of Cardiology* 85, no. 2 (January 15, 2000): 251–5, https://www.ncbi.nlm.nih.gov/pubmed/10955386.

98   Jason A. Gilliland et al., "Linking childhood obesity to the built environment: a multi-level analysis of home and school neighbourhood factors associated with body mass index," *Canadian Journal of Public Health* 103, no. 9 supplement 3 (July 26, 2012): eS15–21, https://www.ncbi.nlm.nih.gov/pubmed/23618083.

99   Meizi He et al., "The influence of local food environments on adolescents' food purchasing behaviors," *International Journal of Environmental Research and Public Health* 9, no. 4 (April 16, 2012): 1458–71, https://www.ncbi.nlm.nih.gov/pmc/articles/PMC3366623/.

100   Where HFCS 42 refers to 42% and HFCS 55 to 55% fructose composition in manufacturing, respectively. HFCS 42 is mainly used for processed foods

and breakfast cereals, whereas HFCS 55 is used mostly for production of soft drinks. "High fructose corn syrup: questions and answers," *US Food and Drug Administration*, https://www.fda.gov/food/food-additives-petitions/high-fructose-corn-syrup-questions-and-answers (accessed March 3, 2017).

101    Vasanti S. Malik and Frank B. Hu, "Fructose and cardiometabolic health: what the evidence from sugar-sweetened beverages tells us," *Journal of the American College of Cardiology* 66, no. 14 (October 6, 2015): 1615–24, https://www.ncbi.nlm.nih.gov/pubmed/26429086.

102    There are multiple complex steps in fructose metabolism:

1. The first step in the metabolism of fructose is the phosphorylation of fructose to fructose 1-phosphate by fructokinase, trapping fructose for metabolism in the liver.

2. Fructose 1-phosphate then undergoes hydrolysis by aldolase B to form dihydroxyacetone phosphate (DHAP) and glyceraldehydes; DHAP can either be isomerized to glyceraldehyde 3-phosphate by triosephosphate isomerase or undergo reduction to glycerol 3-phosphate by glycerol 3-phosphate dehydrogenase.

3. The glyceraldehyde produced may also be converted to glyceraldehyde 3-phosphate by glyceraldehyde kinase or further converted to glycerol 3-phosphate by glycerol 3-phosphate dehydrogenase.

4. The metabolism of fructose at this point yields intermediates in the gluconeogenic pathway leading to glycogen synthesis, but only if there is a need for glycogen synthesis, or as fatty acid and triglyceride synthesis.

5. Once liver glycogen is replenished, the intermediates of fructose metabolism are primarily directed toward triglyceride (or fatty) synthesis.

6. Because of the lack of fasting and abundant access to food, most of the fructose goes directly into the beta oxidation and into the fat cells (adipocytes) for fat storage. Medina Villaamil et al., "Fructose transporter GLUT5 expression in clear renal cell carcinoma," *Oncology Reports* 25, no. 2 (February 2011): 315–23, https://www.ncbi.nlm.nih.gov/pubmed/21165569.

103    Patrick J. Skerrett, "Is fructose bad for you?" *Harvard Health Publishing* (April 21, 2011), https://www.health.harvard.edu/blog/is-fructose-bad-for-you-201104262425.

104    Brandon H. Mai and Liang-Jun Yan, "The negative and detrimental effects of high fructose on the liver, with special reference to metabolic disorders," *Diabetes,*

*Metabolic Syndrome and Obesity* 12 (May 27, 2019): 821–6, https://www.ncbi.nlm.nih.gov/pmc/articles/PMC6549781/.

105   Hyon K. Choi, Walter Willett and Gary Curhan, "Fructose-rich beverages and risk of gout in women," *JAMA* 304, no. 20 (November 24, 2010): 2270–8, https://jamanetwork.com/journals/jama/fullarticle/186958.

106   *Corn Naturally*, http://www.cornnaturally.com/Economics-of-HFCS/price-calculator.aspx (accessed August 15, 2019).

107   Ahmad Esmaillzadeh et al., "Dietary patterns, insulin resistance, and prevalence of the metabolic syndrome in women," *American Journal of Clinical Nutrition* 85, no. 3 (March 2007): 910–8, https://academic.oup.com/ajcn/article/85/3/910/4633067.

108   Neira Sáinz et al., "Leptin resistance and diet-induced obesity: central and peripheral actions of leptin," *Metabolism* 64, no. 1 (January 2015): 35–46, https://www.sciencedirect.com/science/article/abs/pii/S0026049514003096.

109   Miguel A. Lanaspa et al., "High salt intake causes leptin resistance and obesity in mice by stimulating endogenous fructose production and metabolism," *Proceedings of the National Academy of Science of the United States of America* 115, no. 40 (October 2, 2018): E9509, https://www.ncbi.nlm.nih.gov/pmc/articles/PMC6176647/.

110   In a well-controlled animal study, the authors found a significant difference between the groups in 21 bacterial families. These included Akkermansia, SMB53, Proteus, Facklamia, Corynebacterium, Sarcina, Lachnospira, Staphylococcus, 02 d06, Aggregatibacter, Actinomyces, Helicobacter, Turicibacter, Streptococcus, Acinetobacter, Rothia, Aerococcus, Anaerovibrio, Candidatus Arthromitus, Prevotella and Jeotgalicoccus. Out of the identified bacterial genera, they found five bacterial families with trimethylamine-producing capacity: Clostridium, Collinsella, Desulfovibrio, Lactobacillus and Proteus. Klaudia Bielinska et al., "High salt intake increases plasma trimethylamine N-oxide (TMAO) concentration and produces gut dysbiosis in rats," *Nutrition* 54 (October 2018): 33–9, https://www.ncbi.nlm.nih.gov/pubmed/29705499.

111   Cuiting Zhi et al., "Connection between gut microbiome and the development of obesity," *European Journal of Clinical Microbiology and Infectious Diseases* 38, no. 11 (November 2019): 1997–1998, https://www.ncbi.nlm.nih.gov/pubmed/31367997.

112   Myoungsook Lee et al., "Salt induces adipogenesis/lipogenesis and inflammatory adipocytokines secretion in adipocytes," *International Journal of Molecular Science* 20, no. 1 (January 2019):160, https://www.ncbi.nlm.nih.gov/pmc/articles/PMC6337705/.

113   Matt McMillen, "The connection between salt and weight," *WebMD,* May 1, 2017, https://www.webmd.com/diet/obesity/news/20170501/salt-weight-connection (accessed August 15, 2019).

114   "Ghrelin," *You and Your Hormones,* https://www.yourhormones.info/hormones/ghrelin/ (accessed August 15, 2019).

115   Yong Zhang et al., "Elevation of fasting ghrelin in healthy human subjects consuming a high-salt diet: a novel mechanism of obesity?" *Nutrients* 8, no. 6 (May 26, 2016): e323, https://www.ncbi.nlm.nih.gov/pubmed/27240398.

116   Luis Serra-Majem and Inmaculada Bautista-Castaño, "Relationship between bread and obesity," *British Journal of Nutrition* 113, supplement 2 (April 2015): S29–35, https://www.ncbi.nlm.nih.gov/pubmed/26148919.

117   "Obesity update 2017," *OECD,* https://www.oecd.org/els/health-systems/Obesity-Update-2017.pdf (accessed August 15, 2019).

118   "Finland: nutrition, physical activity and obesity," *World Health Organization* (2013), http://www.euro.who.int/__data/assets/pdf_file/0008/243296/Finland-WHO-Country-Profile.pdf?ua=1 (accessed August 15, 2019).

119   The proportion of men and women who were obese dropped from 23.3% in men and 22.8% in women in 2008 to 20.4% in men and 19.0% in women in 2012. This parallels the ongoing salt reduction. In Cyprus, which has the lowest-salt intake in Europe, Eurostat data showed in 2016 an average obesity rate on the island of 14.5%, while in the European Union, it was recorded at 15.9%. Obesity in men is more widespread at 16.3%, with women trailing behind about 3% lower at 12.9%. That is significantly lower than Finland or the European Union, but of course there is also the impact of the Mediterranean diet, a known beneficial factor for longevity.

## Chapter 6: Chronic Kidney Disease and Salt

120   Kris Gunnars, "Intermittent fasting 101—the ultimate beginner's guide," *healthline,* https://www.healthline.com/nutrition/intermittent-fasting-guide (accessed August 19, 2019).

121   Klan Y. Ho et al., "Fasting enhances growth hormone secretion and amplifies the complex rhythms of growth hormone secretion in man," *Journal of Clinical Investigation* 81, no. 4 (April 1988): 968–75, https://www.ncbi.nlm.nih.gov/pmc/articles/PMC329619/.

122   Leonie K. Heilbronn et al., "Alternate-day fasting in nonobese subjects: effects on body weight, body composition, and energy metabolism," *American Journal of*

*Clinical Nutrition* 81, no. 1 (January 1, 2005): 69–73, https://academic.oup.com/ajcn/article/81/1/69/4607679.

123   Intermittent fasting facilitates weight loss and results in an increase of the metabolic rate by 3.6–14.0%. Peter Mansell, Ian W. Fellows and Ian A. Macdonald, "Enhanced thermogenic response to epinephrine after 48-h starvation in humans," *American Journal of Physiology* 258, no. 1 pt 2 (January 1990): r87–93, https://www.ncbi.nlm.nih.gov/pubmed/2405717.

124   Normally only tiny amounts of albumin are present in the urine (depending on age, mostly less than 2.0 mg/mmol creatinine).

125   Arsalan Khaledifar et al., "Association between salt intake and albuminuria in normotensive and hypertensive individuals," *International Journal of Hypertension* v. 2013 (September 19, 2013): 523682, https://www.ncbi.nlm.nih.gov/pmc/articles/PMC3793292/.

126   In that study, there was a significant positive correlation between 24-hour urinary sodium secretion and the level of urine albumin (beta = 0.130, P < 0.001). The amount of salt intake was also significantly associated with urine albumin concentration (beta = 3.969, SE = 1.671, P = 0.018). That study was conducted in 820 individuals. Even after adjusting for other risk factors, this association remained significant. In another study of 1,212 individuals with Type 1 diabetes, higher salt intake (determined by 24-hour urinary sodium excretion) was positively associated with microalbuminuria. Arsalan Khaledifar et al., "Association between salt intake and albuminuria."

127   "Microalbuminuria,"   *Wikipedia,*   https://en.wikipedia.org/wiki/Microalbuminuria (accessed August 17, 2019).

128   Matthew   R.   Weir,   "Dietary   salt,   blood   pressure,   and   microalbuminuria," *Journal   of   Clinical   Hypertension* 6,   no.   11   supplement   3   (November   2004):   23–6,   https://www.researchgate.net/publication/51369299_Dietary_Salt_Blood_Pressure_and_Microalbuminuria.

129   In diabetics, microalbuminuria is the most important biomarker for kidney damage. This is the most devastating complication of diabetes that leads to kidney failure and premature death. Diabetic kidney disease (nephropathy) is characterized by persistent albumin in the urine, elevated blood pressure, relentless decline in kidney function and increased cardiovascular diseases. Microalbuminuria is central to clinical practice to monitor and treat diabetic nephropathy. Microalbuminuria is also a powerful independent predictor for fatal and nonfatal cardiovascular disease in diabetes. Improved blood sugar control, blood pressure reduction (especially using renin-angiotensin-aldosterone-system blockade) and control of other risk factors will reduce the risk of kidney and cardiovascular disease. Hans-Henrik Parving, Frederick Persson and Peter Rossing, "Microalbuminuria: a parameter that has changed

diabetes care," *Diabetes Research and Clinical Practice* 107, no. 1 (January 2015): 1–8, https://www.ncbi.nlm.nih.gov/pubmed/25467616.

130   Leah-Anne M. Ruta et al., "High-salt diet reveals the hypertensive and renal effects of reduced nephron endowment," *American Journal of Physiology Renal Physiology* 298, no. 6 (June 1, 2010): F1384–92, https://journals.physiology.org/doi/full/10.1152/ajprenal.00049.2010.

131   Rebecca C. Berger et al., "Renal effects and underlying molecular mechanisms of long-term salt content diets in spontaneously hypertensive rats," *PLoS One* 10, no. 10 (October 23, 2015): e0141288, https://www.ncbi.nlm.nih.gov/pubmed/26495970.

132   Leif Oxburgh, "Kidney nephron determination," *Annual Review of Cell and Developmental Biology* 34 (October 2018): 427–50, https://www.annualreviews.org/doi/abs/10.1146/annurev-cellbio-100616-060647.

133   Carolyn L. Abitbol and Julie R. Ingelfinger, "Nephron mass and cardiovascular and renal disease risks," *Seminars in Nephrology* 29, no. 4 (July 2009): 445–54, https://www.ncbi.nlm.nih.gov/pubmed/19615565.

134   Prematurity, which is constantly on the rise, partly because of maternal obesity, leads to lower nephron endowment and lifelong consequences. Carolyn L. Abitbol, Marissa Defreitas and José Strauss, "Assessment of kidney function in preterm infants: lifelong implications," *Pediatric Nephrology* 31, no. 12 (December 2016): 2213–22, https://www.researchgate.net/publication/293044411_Assessment_of_kidney_function_in_preterm_infants_lifelong_implications.

135   Matthew Edwards, "The Barker hypothesis," *Handbook of Famine, Starvation, and Nutrient Deprivation* (July 25, 2017): 1–21, https://link.springer.com/referenceworkentry/10.1007%2F978-3-319-40007-5_71-1 (accessed August 18, 2019).

136   "Preterm birth," *World Health Organization* (February 19, 2018), https://www.who.int/news-room/fact-sheets/detail/preterm-birth (accessed August 10, 2019).

137   Li Liu et al., "Global, regional, and national causes of under-5 mortality in 2000–15: an updated systematic analysis with implications for the Sustainable Development Goals," *The Lancet* 388, no. 10063 (November 10, 2016): 3027–35, https://www.thelancet.com/journals/lancet/article/PIIS0140-6736(16)31593-8/fulltext.

138   Mohamed Mohany et al., "A new model for fetal programming: maternal Ramadan-type fasting programs nephrogenesis," *Journal of Developmental Origins of Health and Disease* 9, no. 3 (June 2018): 287–98, https://www.cambridge.org/core/journals/journal-of-developmental-origins-of-health-and-disease/article/new-model-

for-fetal-programming-maternal-ramadantype-fasting-programs-nephrogenesis/
A5EDE4340D9DD1B23D9CA17ED469083C.

139    Nadezda Koleganova, Grzegorz Piecha and Eberhard Ritz, "Prenatal causes of
kidney disease," *Blood Purification* 27, no. 1 (February 2009): 48–52, https://www.
researchgate.net/publication/23939329_Prenatal_Causes_of_Kidney_Disease.

140    Ronit Calderon-Margalit et al., "History of childhood kidney disease and risk of
adult end-stage renal disease," *New England Journal of Medicine* 378, no. 5 (February
2018): 428–438, https://www.nejm.org/doi/full/10.1056/NEJMoa1700993.

141    Julie R. Ingelfinger, "A disturbing legacy of childhood kidney disease," *New
England Journal of Medicine* 378, no. 5 (February 1, 2018): 470–1, https://www.
nejm.org/doi/full/10.1056/NEJMe1716499.

142    Carmen Inés Rodriguez Cuellar et al., "Role of pediatric nephrologists."

143    "Reduce salt intake and maintain health," *State of Israel Ministry of Health*,
https://www.health.gov.il/English/Topics/FoodAndNutrition/Nutrition/Adequate_
nutrition/Na-reduce/Pages/Na-reduce_2.aspx (accessed 18/Aug/2019).

144    Roberto Boero, Angelo Pignataro and Francesco Quarello, "Salt intake and
kidney disease," *Journal of Nephrology* 15, no. 3 (May–June 2002): 225–9, https://
www.ncbi.nlm.nih.gov/pubmed/12113591.

145    Carlo Garofalo et al., "Dietary restriction in chronic kidney disease: a meta-
analysis of randomized clinical trials," *Nutrients* 10, no. 6 (June 2018): E732, https://
www.ncbi.nlm.nih.gov/pmc/articles/PMC6024651/.

146    Emma J. McMahon et al., "A randomized trial of dietary sodium restriction
in CKD," *Journal of the American Society of Nephrology* 24, no. 12 (December 2013):
2096–103, https://jasn.asnjournals.org/content/24/12/2096.

147    Heart failure medications that target sodium excretion are angiotensin II
receptor blocker and neprilysin inhibition.

148    John J. McMurray et al., "Angiotensin-neprilysin inhibition versus enalapril
in heart failure," *New England Journal of Medicine* 371, no. 11 (September 2014):
993–1004, https://www.ncbi.nlm.nih.gov/pubmed/25176015.

149    There is scant data on the epidemiology of heart failure in Finland; however,
a study of 18,346 Finnish men and 19,729 Finnish women showed a clear inverse
correlation between lifestyle patterns and the risk of heart failure. Unfortunately, the
study enrolled patients between 1982 and 2002, so the true value of the population-
wide salt reduction in Finland could not be assessed. By contrast, the cumulative
incidence of end-stage kidney disease has decreased markedly in Finland over the
past five decades since the focus on salt intake became a national priority. Of course,

the causes are multifactorial, but clearly reduced salt intake has contributed to the findings for which Finland should be congratulated. Jaakko Helve et al., "Incidence of end-stage renal disease in patients with type 1 diabetes," *Diabetes Care, American Diabetes Association*, 41, no. 3 (March 2018): 434–9, https://care.diabetesjournals. org/content/41/3/434.

150 According to the 2016 census, Aboriginal peoples in Canada totalled 1,673,785, or 4.9% of the national population. In Canada, the standardized prevalence rate of diabetes is 17.2% of the Indigenous population. The Indigenous population has a higher prevalence of end-stage kidney disease and higher death rates from chronic kidney disease. First Nations people have a higher risk of end-stage renal disease than other groups—the risk of death is 2.6 times higher. "Indigenous peoples in Canada," *Wikipedia*, https://en.wikipedia.org/wiki/Indigenous_peoples_ in_Canada (accessed August 18, 2019). "Type 2 diabetes and Indigenous people," *Diabetes Canada*, https://guidelines.diabetes.ca/cpg/chapter38 (accessed August 18, 2019). Roland Dyck, Ying Jiang and Nathaniel D. Osgood, "The long-term risks of end stage renal disease and mortality among First Nations and non-First Nations people with youth-onset diabetes," *Canadian Journal of Diabetes* 38, no. 4 (August 2014): 237–43, https://www.ncbi.nlm.nih.gov/pubmed/24986804.

## Chapter 7: Dementia and Salt

151 "Lewy body dementia," *Mayo Clinic*, https://www.mayoclinic.org/diseases-conditions/lewy-body-dementia/symptoms-causes/syc-20352025 (accessed August 20, 2019).

152 "Frontotemporal dementia," *Mayo Clinic*, https://www.mayoclinic.org/ diseases-conditions/frontotemporal-dementia/symptoms-causes/syc-20354737 (accessed August 20, 2019).

153 "Dementia," *Wikipedia*, https://en.wikipedia.org/wiki/Dementia (accessed August 19, 2019).

154 Antonio Lobo et al., "Prevalence of dementia and major subtypes in Europe: a collaborative study of population-based cohorts. Neurologic Diseases in the Elderly Research Group," *Neurology* 54, no. 11 supplement 5 (2000): S4–9, https://www. ncbi.nlm.nih.gov/pubmed/10854355.

155 "Creutzfeldt-Jakob disease," *Mayo Clinic*, https://www.mayoclinic.org/ diseases-conditions/creutzfeldt-jakob-disease/symptoms-causes/syc-20371226 (accessed August 20, 2019).

156 "Understanding Parkinson's," *Parkinson Canada*, https://www.parkinson.ca/ about-parkinsons/understanding-parkinsons/ (accessed August 20, 2019).

157 "Huntington's disease," *Mayo Clinic*, https://www.mayoclinic.org/diseases-conditions/huntingtons-disease/symptoms-causes/syc-20356117 (accessed August 20, 2019).

158 "Dementia," *Wikipedia.*

159 "Latest information and statistics," *Alzheimer Society Canada*, https://alzheimer.ca/en/Home/Get-involved/Advocacy/Latest-info-stats (accessed August 19, 2019).

160 "Population projections for Canada, provinces and territories," *Statistics Canada*, https://www150.statcan.gc.ca/n1/pub/91-520-x/2010001/aftertoc-apre-stdm1-eng.htm (accessed August 19, 2019).

161 Giuseppe Faraco et al., "Dietary salt promotes neurovascular and cognitive dysfunction through a gut-initiated TH17 response," *Nature Neuroscience* 21, no. 2 (January 15, 2018): 240–9, https://www.nature.com/articles/s41593-017-0059-z.

162 Seung Min Jung et al., "Sodium chloride aggravates arthritis via Th17 polarization," *Yonsei Medical Journal* 60, no. 1 (January 2019): 88–97, https://www.ncbi.nlm.nih.gov/pmc/articles/PMC6298894/.

163 Saeid Taheri et al., "High-sodium diet has opposing effects on mean arterial blood pressure and cerebral perfusion in a transgenic mouse model of Alzheimer's disease," *Journal of Alzheimer's Disease* 54, no. 3 (October 4, 2016): 1061–72, https://www.ncbi.nlm.nih.gov/pubmed/27567835.

164 The mice were fed a diet that contained salt levels equivalent to more than one teaspoon per day for humans—the recommendation by the US Department of Agriculture hovers around three-quarters of a teaspoon per day, although we have shown that the average intake is about twice that. Stimulated by high-salt diet, these cells produce high levels of circulating plasma interleukin 17 (IL-17), which is a pro-inflammatory cytokine. After binding to the corresponding IL-17 receptors, IL-17 activates several signalling cascades that, in turn, lead to the induction of chemokines. Acting as chemo-attractants, these chemokines recruit immune cells, such as monocytes and neutrophils to the site of inflammation. The end effect is both an allergic response and ultimately tissue scarring. "Interleukin 17," *Wikipedia*, https://en.wikipedia.org/wiki/Interleukin_17 (accessed August 20, 2019).

165 Francesca Pistollato et al., "Associations between sleep, cortisol regulation, and diet: possible implications for the risk of Alzheimer disease," *Advances in Nutrition* 7, no. 4 (July 2016): 679–89, https://www.ncbi.nlm.nih.gov/pubmed/27422503.

166 *Alzheimer's association*, https://www.alzheimersanddementia.com/article/S1552-5260(11)01858-9/pdf (accessed August 20, 2019).

167    Laura A. Warren et al., "Prevalence and incidence of dementia among indigenous populations: a systematic review," *International Psychogeriatrics* 27, no. 12 (December 2015): 1959–70, https://www.ncbi.nlm.nih.gov/pubmed/26088474.

## Chapter 8: Vision and Salt

168    Visual impairment of 5.7% (95% CI 5.4–6.0). Rumaisa Aljied et al., "Prevalence and determinants of visual impairment in Canada: cross-sectional data from the Canadian Longitudinal Study on Aging," *Canadian Journal of Ophthalmology* 53, no. 3 (June 2018): 291–7, https://www.canadianjournalofophthalmology.ca/article/S0008-4182(17)31135-3/fulltext.

169    "Cataract," *Wikipedia*, https://en.wikipedia.org/wiki/Cataract (accessed August 21, 2019).

170    "Global data on visual impairments 2010," *World Health Organization* (2012): 6, https://www.who.int/blindness/GLOBALDATAFINALforweb.pdf.

171    "Priority eye diseases," *World Health Organization*, https://www.who.int/blindness/causes/priority/en/index1.html (accessed August 21, 2019).

172    "Cataract tables," *National Eye Institute*, https://www.nei.nih.gov/learn-about-eye-health/resources-for-health-educators/eye-health-data-and-statistics/cataract-data-and-statistics/cataract-tables (accessed August 21, 2019).

173    In a well-conducted European literature review, Prokofyeva et al reported that the risk for cataracts was significantly increased by former smoking (3.75-fold risk), current smoking (2.34-fold risk), asthma or chronic bronchitis (2.04-fold risk), and cardiovascular disease (1.96-fold risk). Some drugs may cause cataracts. The study states: "Cataract was more common in patients taking chlorpromazine during 90 days with a dosage 300 mg or more (8.8-fold risk) and corticosteroids over 5 years (3.25-fold risk) in a daily dose greater than 1600 mg (1.69-fold risk). Intake of a multivitamin/mineral formulation (2.0-fold risk) or corticosteroids (2.12-fold risk) also increased the risk of cataract." Now, this is confusing because vitamin supplementation is normally seen as protective. There may have been a bias because people at risk may be more prone to taking supplements. The association with vitamin supplement intake is interesting and may be an important strategy to lower the incidence of cataract. Elena Prokofyeva, Alfred Wegener and Eberhart Zrenner, "Cataract prevalence and prevention in Europe: a literature review," *Acta Ophthalmologica* 91, no. 5 (August 2013): 395–405, https://www.ncbi.nlm.nih.gov/pubmed/22715900.

174    Julie A. Mares-Perlman et al., "Vitamin supplement use and incident cataracts in a population-based study," *Archives of Ophthalmology* 118, no. 11 (November 2000): 1556–63, https://www.ncbi.nlm.nih.gov/pubmed/11074813.

175   Suqian Wu and Jianjiang Xu, "Incidence and risk factors for post-penetrating keratoplasty glaucoma: A systematic review and meta-analysis," *PLoS One* 12, no. 4 (April 21, 2017): e0176261, https://www.ncbi.nlm.nih.gov/pubmed/28430806.

176   On logistic regression, a linear increase of cataract prevalence with salt intake was found, which was highly significant across quartiles. In the adjusted analysis, there was a 1.13-fold increase with each doubling of the urinary sodium to creatinine ratio. Ekaterina Yonova-Doing et al., "Genetic and dietary factors influencing the progression of nuclear cataract," *Ophthalmology* 123, no. 6 (June 2016): 1237–44, https://www.ncbi.nlm.nih.gov/pmc/articles/PMC4882156/.

177   High sodium intake is defined as a urinary sodium to creatinine ratio greater than 16.4 mmol/mmol. Jeong Hun Bae et al., "Sodium intake and socio-economic status as risk factors for development of age-related cataracts: the Korea National Health and Nutrition Examination Survey," *PLoS One* 10, no. 8 (2015): e0136218, https://journals.plos.org/plosone/article/file?id=10.1371/journal.pone.0136218&type=printable.

178   Robert G. Cumming, Paul Mitchell and Wayne Smith, "Dietary sodium intake and cataract: the Blue Mountains Eye Study," *American Journal of Epidemiology* 151, no. 6 (March 15, 2000): 624–6, https://academic.oup.com/aje/article/151/6/624/113776.

179   An animal study reported changes in ion transport and electrolyte imbalance in the lenses of rats on a high-salt diet. Nalin J. Unakar and Margaret Johnson, "Lenticular alterations in hypertensive rats," *Experimental Eye Research* 59, no. 6 (December 1994): 645–52, https://www.ncbi.nlm.nih.gov/pubmed/7698259. This particular rat model represents hypertensive rats, limiting its generalizability. However, more than half of the human population over age 40 is hypertensive. In another rat model, increased dietary sodium chloride intake influenced lens transport properties, unrelated to blood pressure levels. Estela S. Estapé et al., "Increased dietary NaCl intake influences lens transport properties in Sprague-Dawley rats," *Current Eye Research* 14, no. 2 (February 1995): 159–62, https://www.ncbi.nlm.nih.gov/pubmed/7768108.

180   "A comprehensive global monitoring framework," WHO.

181   Matin Ghanavati et al., "Healthy eating index in patients with cataract: a case-control study," *Iranian Red Crescent Medical Journal* 17, no. 10 (October 2015):e22490, https://www.ncbi.nlm.nih.gov/pmc/articles/PMC4640062/.

182   Liz Segre, "What does cataract surgery cost?" *All About Vision*, https://www.all-aboutvision.com/conditions/cataract-surgery-cost.htm (accessed August 21, 2019).

183   "Cataracts surgery in Ontario," *Eye Physicians and Surgeons of Ontario*, https:// www.epso.ca/frequently-asked-questions/cataract-surgery-in-ontario-2/   (accessed August 21, 2019).

184   Hugh R. Taylor, Mariateresa Pezzullo and Jill Keeffe, "The economic impact and cost of visual impairment in Australia," *British Journal of Ophthalmology* 90, no. 3 (March 2006): 272–5, https://www.ncbi.nlm.nih.gov/pmc/articles/PMC1856946/.

185   "Age-related macular degeneration," *National Eye Institute* (June 2015), https://www.nei.nih.gov/learn-about-eye-health/eye-conditions-and-diseases/age-related-macular-degeneration (accessed August 21, 2019).

186   "Sodium food sources in the Canadian diet."

187   Jennifer R. Evans and John G. Lawrenson, "Antioxidant vitamin and mineral supplements to prevent the development of age-related macular degeneration," *Cochrane Database of Systematic Reviews* 7 (July 2017): CD000253, https://www. cochrane.org/CD000253/EYES_antioxidant-vitamin-and-mineral-supplements-prevent-development-age-related-macular-degeneration-amd.

188   The molecular mechanism appears to be related to certain growth factors in the blood that are being upregulated when there is increased osmolality. High osmolality also induces expression of aquaporin-5, a water channel implicated in trans-epithelial water transport. Andreas Bringmann et al., "Intake of dietary salt and drinking water: implications for the development of age-related macular degeneration," *Molecular Vision* 22 (December 22, 2016): 1437–54, https://www.ncbi.nlm. nih.gov/pubmed/28031693.

## Chapter 9: Cardiovascular Health and Salt

189   In an animal model, Matsushita et al demonstrated that accumulation of sodium in water is associated with aneurysm formation in the brain. Nobuhisa Matsushita et al., "Increase in body Na+/water ratio is associated with cerebral aneurysm formation in oophorectomized rats," *Hypertension* 60, no. 5 (November 2012). 1309–15, https://www.ncbi.nlm.nih.gov/pubmed/23045463.

190   A meta-analysis of 185 studies that examined the benefits of a sodium diet from an average sodium intake of 201 mmol/day (high intake) to 66 mmol/day (recommended intake). "LDL and HDL: 'bad' and 'good' cholesterol," *Centers for Disease Control and Prevention CDC*, https://www.cdc.gov/cholesterol/ldl_hdl.htm (accessed September 11, 2017).

191   "Low-density lipoprotein," *Wikipedia*, https://en.wikipedia.org/wiki/Low-density_lipoprotein (accessed August 22, 2019).

192  LDL is calculated using the Friedewald formula. This formula is known to perform poorly in the setting of elevated triglycerides or very high cholesterol concentrations. We are therefore not even certain that the LDL determinations are correct. R. Sam Niedbala et al., "Estimation of low-density lipoprotein by the Friedewald formula and by electrophoresis compared," *Clinical Chemistry* 31, no. 10 (October 1985): 1762–3, https://academic.oup.com/clinchem/article/31/10/1762/5651988.

193  There was no dose-response of sodium intake on serum lipids or the cholesterol ratio in either diet. In that study, changes in salt intake over the range of 50–150 mmol per day did not affect blood lipid concentrations. David W. Harsha et al., "Effect of dietary sodium intake on blood lipids: results from the DASH–sodium trial," *Hypertension* 43, no. 2 (January 5, 2004): 393–8, https://www.ahajournals.org/doi/full/10.1161/01.HYP.0000113046.83819.a2.

194  In a recent study that controlled for obesity of 3,294 adults, associations were highly affected by adjustment for obesity. Obesity significantly affects cholesterol levels. Adipose (fat) tissue has high lipolytic activity, releasing fatty acids in the portal (liver) and body circulations. In the liver, fatty acids affect lipid metabolism and stimulate cholesterol synthesis, which is associated with the production of proinflammatory and proatherogenic cytokines. Femke Taverne et al. "Abdominal obesity, insulin resistance, metabolic syndrome and cholesterol homeostasis," *PharmaNutrition* 1, no. 4 (2013): 130–6, https://www.sciencedirect.com/science/article/pii/S221343441300039X.

195  Betina H. Thuesen et al., "Estimated daily salt intake in relation to blood pressure and blood lipids: the role of obesity," *European Journal of Preventive Cardiology* 22, no. 12 (December 2015): 1567–74, https://www.ncbi.nlm.nih.gov/pubmed/25281483.

196  Lorena Allemandi et al., "Sodium content in processed foods in Argentina."

197  This is based on a study of 12,267 persons. At a 14.8-year follow-up, increased dietary sodium intake increased all-cause mortality by 20% per 1,000 mg per day of increased dietary sodium, whereas increased dietary potassium decreased all-cause mortality by 20% per 1,000 mg per day of increased dietary potassium. Quanhe Yang et al., "Sodium and potassium intake and mortality among US adults: prospective data from the Third National Health and Nutrition Examination Survey," *Archives of Internal Medicine* 171 (2011): 1183–91, https://www.ncbi.nlm.nih.gov/pubmed/21747015.

198  Heikki Karppanen and Eero Mervaala, "Sodium intake and hypertension," *Progress in Cardiovascular Diseases* 49, no. 2 (September–October 2006): 59–75, https://www.ncbi.nlm.nih.gov/pubmed/17046432.

199   Edward D. Frohlich and Dinko Susic, "Sodium and its multiorgan targets," *Circulation* 124 (October 25, 2011): 1882–5, https://www.ahajournals.org/doi/full/10.1161/circulationaha.111.029371.

200   Hsing-Yi Chang et al. "Effect of potassium-enriched salt on cardiovascular mortality and medical expenses of elderly men," *American Journal of Clinical Nutrition* 83, no. 6 (June 2006): 1289–96, https://www.ncbi.nlm.nih.gov/pubmed/16762939.

201   Paul K. Whelton, "Sodium, potassium, blood pressure, and cardiovascular disease in humans," *Current Hypertension Reports* 16, no. 8 (August 2014): 465, https://www.ncbi.nlm.nih.gov/pubmed/24924995.

202   "Heart failure," *Mayo Clinic*, https://www.mayoclinic.org/diseases-conditions/heart-failure/symptoms-causes/syc-20373142 (accessed August 23, 2019).

203   ER Heerdink et al., "NSAIDs associated with increased risk of congestive heart failure in elderly patients taking diuretics," *Archives of Internal Medicine* 158, no. 10 (May 25, 1998): 1108–12, https://www.ncbi.nlm.nih.gov/pubmed/9605782.

204   Eric Wooltorton, "Rosiglitazone (Avandia) and pioglitazone (Actos) and heart failure," *CMAJ* 166, no. 2 (January 22, 2002): 219, http://www.cmaj.ca/content/166/2/219, (accessed August 23, 2019).

205   ER Heerdink et al., "NSAIDs associated with increased risk of congestive heart failure."

## Chapter 10: Why Was the Finnish Salt Campaign so Effective?

206   Emily Willingham, "Finland's bold push to change the heart health of a nation," *Knowable Magazine* (July 3, 2018), https://www.knowablemagazine.org/article/health-disease/2018/finlands-bold-push-change-heart-health-nation (accessed September 4, 2019).

207   Emily Willingham, "Finland's bold push."

208   Katja Borodulin et al., "Cohort profile: the National FINRISK Study," *International Journal of Epidemiology* 47, no. 3 (June 2018): 696–6i, https://doi.org/10.1093/ije/dyx239.

209   Pekka Jousilahti et al., "40-year CHD mortality trends and the role of risk factors in mortality decline: the North Karelia Project experience," *Global Heart* 11, no. 2 (June 2016): 207–12, https://www.ncbi.nlm.nih.gov/pubmed/27242088.

210   For example, "among the working aged, total cholesterol levels declined from 6.77 mmol/L to 5.44 mmol/L during 1972–2012 in North Karelian men, and

coronary heart disease mortality decreased by 82% (from 643 to 118 per 100,000) among men and by 84% (from 114 to 17 per 100,000) among women." These changes were profound. Erkki Vartiainen et al., "Do changes in cardiovascular risk factors explain changes in mortality from stroke in Finland?" *BMJ* 310, no. 6984 (April 8, 1995): 901–4, https://www.ncbi.nlm.nih.gov/pmc/articles/PMC2549289/.

211   "Food and nutrition," *Government of Canada*, https://food-guide.canada.ca/en/ (accessed September 4, 2019).

212   "Current smoking prevalence," *Tobacco Use in Canada*, https://uwaterloo.ca/tobacco-use-canada/adult-tobacco-use/smoking-canada/current-smoking-prevalence (accessed September 4, 2019).

213   Francesco Cappuccio et al., "Policy options to reduce population salt intake," *BMJ* 343 (August 2011): d4995, https://www.bmj.com/content/343/bmj.d4995.

214   Sara Chodosh, "The CDC knows why U.S. life expectancy keeps dropping."

215   Lorena Allemandi et al., "Sodium content in processed foods in Argentina."

216   Francesco P. Cappuccio, "Sodium and potassium intake: facts, issues and controversies, nutritional and public health perspectives," Official Lectures, *Warwick Medical School*, https://warwick.ac.uk/fac/sci/med/staff/cappuccio/officiallectures/ (accessed September 4, 2019).

## Chapter 11: Potential Savings

217   "Ontario patients wait longer for cataract surgery, while waits for other priority procedures remain stable," *Canadian Institute for Health Information*, https://www.newswire.ca/news-releases/ontario-patients-wait-longer-for-cataract-surgery-while-waits-for-other-priority-procedures-remain-stable-617267253.html (accessed September 5, 2019).

218   Jean-Eric Tarride et al., "A review of the cost of cardiovascular disease," *Canadian Journal of Cardiology* 25, no. 6 (June 2009): e195–202, https://www.ncbi.nlm.nih.gov/pubmed/19536390.

219   "How to reduce heart disease by 75%," *Pritikin Longevity Center and Spa*, https://www.pritikin.com/your-health/health-benefits/reverse-heart-disease/252-heart-disease-deaths-plunge-75.html (accessed September 7, 2019).

220   Ben Chan and Bill Hayes, "Cost of stroke in Ontario, 1994/95," *Canadian Medical Association* 159, supplement 6 (September 22, 1998), http://www.cmaj.ca/content/cmaj/suppl/2002/04/04/159.6.DC1/S2.pdf (accessed September 7, 2019).

221    "Canada: inflation rate from 1984 to 2024," *Statista*, https://www.statista.com/statistics/271247/inflation-rate-in-canada/ (accessed September 6, 2019).

222    "2019–20 first quarter finances," *Ontario Ministry of Finance*, https://www.fin.gov.on.ca/en/budget/finances/2019/ofin19_1.html (accessed September 7, 2019).

223    Jordan Whitehouse, "Spare some salt? The rock salt shortage of 2018," *Horticultural Trades Association*, https://horttrades.com/spare-some-salt-the-rock-salt-shortage-of-2018 (accessed September 7, 2019).

224    Sobhi Girgis et al., "A one-quarter reduction in the salt content of bread can be made without detection," *European Journal of Clinical Nutrition* 57, no. 4 (April 2003): 616–20, https://www.ncbi.nlm.nih.gov/pubmed/12700625.

225    Kirsten Bibbins-Domingo et al., "Projected effect of dietary salt reductions on future cardiovascular disease," *New England Journal of Medicine* 362, no. 7 (February 2010): 590–9, https://www.ncbi.nlm.nih.gov/pubmed/20089957.

226    Lawrence Appel and Cheryl Anderson, "Compelling evidence for public health action to reduce salt intake," *New England Journal of Medicine* 362, no. 7 (February 2010): 650–2, https://www.nejm.org/doi/full/10.1056/NEJMe0910352.

## Chapter 12: Summary and Conclusions

227    The pharmaceutical industry has realized that the times of blockbuster drugs like Viagra or statins are over, and now they've discovered rare diseases as opportunities for high-cost drugs. Less than 1% of the Canadian population accounts for 42% of patented medicine sales, and the costs are rising at a staggering rate. Between 2006 and 2017, the number of medicines in Canada with an annual per beneficiary cost of at least $10,000 increased by over 200% and now account for 42% of patented medicine sale (fig. 32). Orphan drugs (drugs for rare diseases) are increasingly dominating the market and account for nearly half of new launches. While it is good that pharmaceutical companies are focusing on rare diseases and developing proper drugs for these conditions, the costs are often outrageous. More than 25% of new drugs that were licensed in 2016 or 2017 were for cancer therapy, averaging $13,700 for a 28-day treatment. Even more expensive is the drug eculizumab, a complement cascade inhibitor, which has an indication for two ultra-rare diseases. It used to be priced at up to $700,000 per year. Subsequently, Alexion, the company making eculizumab, was ordered to lower the price. Enzyme replacement therapy for rare metabolic diseases may be equally expensive. Don't get me wrong, I support the development of drugs for rare diseases, however, the pricing has to be reasonable. Furthermore, this is just one element of the rising health care costs. Elena Lungu, "What is the 'expense' for expensive drugs for rare diseases?" presented at the CADTH Symposium, Patented Medicine Prices Review Board, *Government of Canada* (April

2019), http://www.pmprb-cepmb.gc.ca/view.asp?ccid=1461&lang=en (accessed July 8, 2019).

228   "Ounce of prevention, pound of cure," *University of Cambridge* (October 9, 2012), https://www.cam.ac.uk/research/news/ounce-of-prevention-pound-of-cure (accessed September 8, 2019).

229   Pam Belluck, "Children's life expectancy being cut short by obesity," *New York Times* (March 17, 2005), https://www.nytimes.com/2005/03/17/health/childrens-life-expectancy-being-cut-short-by-obesity.html (accessed September 8, 2019).

## List of picture credits

**Figure 2:** *Source*: Lorena Allemandi et al., "Sodium content in processed foods in Argentina: compliance with the national law," Cardiovascular Diagnosis and Therapy 5, no. 3, June 2015, https://www.ncbi.nlm.nih.gov/pmc/articles/PMC4451319/.

**Figure 3:** *Source*: "Information within the nutrition facts table: mandatory information," Canadian Food Inspection Agency, Government of Canada, http://www.inspection.gc.ca/food/requirements-and-guidance/labelling/industry/nutrition-labelling/nutrition-facts-table/eng/1389198568400/1389198597278?chap=1.

**Figure   7:**   *Source*:   Bjorn   Lemmer's   2009   Chronobiology   article, "Discoveries of rhythms in human biological functions: a historical review," https://www.researchgate.net/publication/26790239_Discoveries_of_Rhythms_in_Human_Biological_Functions_A_Historical_Review/figures?lo=1.

**Figure   8:** *Source*: Uwe Diegel, "The man behind the science of blood pressure," Linked   in   (March   24,   2018),   https://www.linkedin.com/pulse/man-behind-science-blood-pressure-uwe-diegel/

**Figure   9:**   *Source*:      Dylan   Collins,   "Doctors   botch   blood   pressure   readings   more   often   than   you   think," Vox   (July   3,   2018),   https://www.vox.com/science-and-health/2018/7/3/17510132/new-blood-pressure-guidelines-ranges-hypertension.

**Figure 10:** *Source*: https://www.shutterstock.com/search/hip+replacement.

**Figure 11:** *Source*: "Does osteoporosis run in your family?" Genomics and Precision Health, Centers for Disease Control and Prevention, https://www.cdc.gov/genomics/disease/osteoporosis.htm?CDC_AA_refVal=https%3A%2F%2Fwww.cdc.gov%2Ffeatures%2Fosteoporosis%2Findex.html.

**Figure 12:** *Source*: Courtesy of the Mayo Foundation for Medical Education and Research.

**Figure 13:** *Source*: Paul D. Miller, "Controversial issues in bone density," in Principles of Bone Biology, 3rd edition (2008), ScienceDirect, https://www.sciencedirect.com/topics/medicine-and-dentistry/bone-mass.

**Figure 14:** *Source*: Osteoporosis," World Action on Salt and Health, http://www.worldactiononsalt.com/salthealth/factsheets/osteoporosis/.

**Figure 16:** *Source*: graph of "Congestive heart failure lung x-ray" Wikimedia Commons, https://commons.wikimedia.org/w/index.php?sort=relevance&search=congestive+heart+failure&title=Special:Search&profile=advanced&fulltext=1&advancedSearch-current=%7B%7D&ns0=1&ns6=1&ns12=1&ns14=1&ns100=1&ns106=1#/media/File:Congestive_heart_failure_x-ray.png.

**Figure 17:** *Source*: Delphi234, graph of "Adult female obesity 20–74 in the United States," Wikipedia, https://commons.wikimedia.org/w/index.php?curid=50288259.

**Figure 18:** *Source*: Delphi234, graph of "Adult male obesity 20-74 in the United States," Wikipedia, https://commons.wikimedia.org/w/index.php?curid=502882560

**Figure 20:** *Source*: "Scientific opinion on the substantiation of health claims related to fructose and reduction of post-prandial glycaemic responses (ID 558) pursuant to Article 13(1) of Regulation (EC) No 1924/2006," European Food Safety Authority Journal 9, no. 6 (June 30, 2011): 2223, https://efsa.onlinelibrary.wiley.com/doi/pdf/10.2903/j.efsa.2011.2223.

**Figure 21:** *Source*: Illustration from "Anatomy and physiology," from Connexions (June 19, 2013), Wikimedia Commons, https://commons.wikimedia.org/w/index.php?curid=30148542.

**Figure 23:** *Source*: Launer Fratiglioni et al., "Incidence of dementia and major subtypes in Europe: a collaborative study of population-based cohorts. Neurologic diseases in the elderly research group," Neurology 54, no. 11 supplement 5 (2000): S10–15, https://www.ncbi.nlm.nih.gov/pubmed/10854355.

**Figure 24:** *Source*: "Causes of death in 2017," Statistics Finland, http://www.stat.fi/til/ksyyt/2017/ksyyt_2017_2018-12-17_kat_001_en.html (accessed August 19, 2019).

**Figure 25:** *Source*: "Age-standardized mortality rates for dementia, by sex, Canada, 2000 and 2017," Statistics Canada, https://www150.statcan.gc.ca/n1/daily-quotidien/190530/cg-c004-png-eng.htm (accessed August 19, 2019).

**Figure 26:** *Source*: "Diagrammatic section through the eyeball," from "Eye," Encyclopaedia Britannica 10 (1911), Wikimedia Commons, https://commons.

wikimedia.org/wiki/File:EB1911_Eye_-_Fig._1.%E2%80%94Diagrammatic_Section_through_the_Eyeball.jpg, (August 21, 2019).

**Figure 27:** *Source*: "Cataract," Wikipedia, https://en.wikipedia.org/wiki/Cataract#cite_note-WHO2014-3 (accessed 21-Aug-2019).

**Figure 28:** *Source*: National Eye Institute, National Institutes of Health Ref#: EDA2.

**Figure 29:** *Source*: "Congestive heart failure x-ray," from Public Health Image Library (1978), Wikimedia Commons, https://commons.wikimedia.org/wiki/File:Congestive_heart_failure_x-ray.png

# About the Author

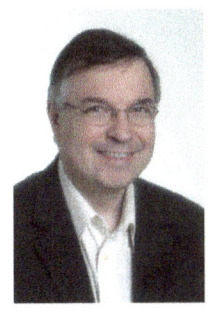

Guido Filler is professor of paediatrics at Western University in London, Ontario, with cross-appointments to medicine and pathology and laboratory medicine. His area of expertise is nephrology. He is also a clinical pharmacologist. He served as chair/chief of the department of paediatrics from 2006-2016. Dr. Filler is a prolific author with over 300 publications in PubMed as well as one book entitled "Becoming a successful scholar" and multiple book chapters. He is a world expert for the measurement of renal function. He has also extensively studied drug disposition in children and youth. Driven by the surge of paediatric patients with kidney stones, he recently expanded his research to this area. The current book originated from that research, which demonstrated the profound impact of our high salt diet on kidney stones. As a system thinker, he provides a solution to the growing incidence of non-communicable diseases.

www.ingramcontent.com/pod-product-compliance
Lightning Source LLC
Chambersburg PA
CBHW041107280526
45792CB00010B/2330